Poisons in Your Food

ALSO BY THE AUTHOR

Beware of the Food You Eat
How to Reduce Your Medical Bills
Ageless Aging
Cancer-Causing Agents
A Consumer's Dictionary of Cosmetic Ingredients
A Consumer's Dictionary of Food Additives

Poisons in Your Food

NEW, REVISED, AND UPDATED EDITION

The Dangers You Face and What You Can Do About Them

RUTH WINTER, M.S.

Crown Publishers, Inc., New York

Published by Crown Publishers, Inc., 201 East 50th Street, New York, New York 10022. Member of the Crown Publishing Group.

CROWN is a trademark of Crown Publishers, Inc.

Manufactured in the United States of America

Library of Congress Cataloging-in-Publication Data

Winter, Ruth, 1930–
    Poisons in your food: the dangers you face and what you can do about them / by Ruth Winter.—New, rev., and updated ed., 1st ed.
        p.   cm.
    1. Food adulteration and inspection.   2. Food contamination.
I. Title.
TX533.W55   1990
641'.31—dc20   89-70833
                                                                    CIP

ISBN 0-517-57681-3

10 9 8 7 6 5 4 3 2 1

Revised Edition

Contents

Introduction

This book is unique!

I researched and wrote the first edition of *Poisons in Your Food* in the late 1960s when I was a young newspaper science editor and the mother of small children.

I discovered at the time that there were:

- Antibiotics, in animal feed, that affected humans who ate meat and drank milk.
- Dangerous pesticide residues in our food.
- Additives in our meals that could cause cancer.
- Drinking waters polluted with industrial wastes.
- Foodborne illnesses that were common, could be lethal, but were often unrecognized and unreported.

Before I researched the first edition of *Poisons in Your Food*, I thought that government inspectors looked over the shoulders of food manufacturers and vendors all along the line. When I discovered nothing could be further from the truth, I pointed out the inadequacies in our food inspection systems. After *Poisons in Your Food* was initially published, I was described as "a nut among the berries" and the book as "sensational," "hysterical," or "fictional."

Today, I am a grandmother and the author of twenty-three other books and hundreds of newspaper and magazine articles about developments in science and health.

I have had the unusual privilege of being able to research anew the same subjects that I investigated more than twenty years ago.

I have lived to see such conservative organizations as the American Cancer Society and the National Cancer Institute expound upon the links between cancer and diet. Today the American Heart Association and the National Heart Institute are leading the battle to have food processors lower fat and salt in foods. The National Academy of Sciences, the Environmental Protection Agency, the General Accounting Office, and other government agencies are now citing flaws in our ability to protect food and water from pesticides, nitrates, and other pollutants, flaws about which I reported more than twenty years ago.

As you will read in this book, the Food and Drug Administration and the National Academy of Sciences admit much is unknown about the more than three thousand chemicals deliberately or inadvertently added to our food.

United States Centers for Disease Control experts maintain that those foodborne illnesses reported represent just a small percentage of the cases that actually occur.

In researching this new edition, I have found that during the past twenty years, some things have gotten better, some have gotten worse, and, frustratingly, many things have remained the same.

The purpose of this book is, as it was when the first edition appeared, to convince you that *not everything causes cancer—that not everything you eat is bad for you!*

The aim of this book is to describe the situation and to educate you about your choices. *You can choose a healthier diet!* You can, by the power of your pocketbook, make food manufacturers and vendors provide healthier selections at the supermarket and in the restaurant. They want to sell their products to you. They are, therefore, exquisitely sensitive to your desires.

You can, by your own knowledge, protect yourself and your family from a great deal of foodborne and waterborne illness. If you are pregnant or have small children, or if you are elderly or have a weakened immune system, information in this book may prevent serious illness and even death.

You cannot do anything about your heredity or your taxes, but you do have the power to choose and handle your food and water wisely.

Poisons in Your Food

1 ⌐ Guess What You Just Ate!

When *Poisons in Your Food* was first published in 1969, I wrote:

> When you sit down to eat a meal in your own home or in one of the 540,000 eating and drinking places in the United States, you take it for granted that the food is wholesome and nutritious. Unless you have access to special knowledge— medical data, reports of qualified investigators, and findings behind the "vital statistics"—it may not occur to you that it is now impossible for you to eat an ordinary meal, or to give a child milk from a bottle, can, carton, or breast, that is not contaminated with pesticides.[1] The sausages, ham, hamburgers, or hot dogs you eat can be filled with hog blood, cereal, lungs, nitrite, water, detergents, and/or sodium sulfite.[2] Even a baby's diet can be dangerous.
>
> The bread you put in your mouth daily is literally embalmed to keep it feeling soft and fresh long after it isn't,[3] and the dessert you eat may be colored with a cancer-causing agent.[4]

More than twenty years later, there are now 720,000 food-service establishments,[5] but what I wrote in 1969 holds true.

- Ten pesticides proven to cause cancer are still leaving residues in raw and processed foods and in breast milk.[6]

- Deaths from "hidden additives" such as sulfites and peanut oil in foods are still occurring.[7]
- We are still endangering our children and theirs with toxic residues in water and food.[8, 9]
- Illnesses from bacterial, viral, and chemical contaminants in food are increasing.[10]

Have you had a case of "intestinal flu" and/or diarrhea this year? Chances are that you have.

Frank Young, M.D., Ph.D., commissioner of the United States Food and Drug Administration (FDA), said in 1988, "Unfortunately, microbial contamination and outbreaks of food-borne illness have continued at an alarming rate. According to estimates by our own FDA scientists, between 21 million and 81 million cases of food-borne diarrheal disease occur annually in the United States."[11]

The Centers for Disease Control (CDC), understaffed and overburdened by the AIDS epidemic, has started reporting foodborne illnesses every five years instead of every year and at the time of this writing are still far behind schedule. Ironically, AIDS victims and others with weakened immune systems are the most vulnerable to foodborne illnesses and may succumb to "intestinal upsets" that would not be fatal to healthy, young adults.

The CDC takes reports from state health departments, not individuals; but did you report to *your* health department your latest bout of stomach upset brought on by "something" you ate?

Most of the time foodborne illnesses are not reported because:

- The discomfort may be self-limiting and not require medical attention.
- The illness, although it does require medical attention, is not recognized by either the victim or the physician as being related to food.

Do you assume that the food you eat at home or in a restaurant has been inspected?

Do you know that most foods from catering establishments, processing plants that sell in one state only, and vending machines are almost never inspected?[12]

Do you know that less than 1 percent of domestic and imported foods are checked for pesticides?

It takes twenty-eight days for the FDA to test and process a sample, and the food is usually sold and eaten by the time the results are known.[13]

When I wrote the first edition of *Poisons in Your Food* in 1969, I pointed out that approximately 60 percent of all fish eaten in the United States originated in foreign countries, a number of which had poor sanitary practices and fish-storage conditions. I noted that only 5 percent of such imports were inspected by the U.S. Food and Drug Administration. At that time, the United States had forty-two hundred fish-processing plants, 75,000 fishing vessels, and sixty-two inspectors from the U.S. Bureau of Fisheries. These inspectors checked forty fish-processing plants, and then only at the request and expense of the processors. It was brought out at the 1969 Senate hearings on fish inspection that 6,273 trained persons would be required to adequately inspect American fish products.[14]

The situation is no better today. We are second only to Japan in the importation of fish—three billion pounds a year.[15] Despite the recognized pollution of our waters and the efforts of consumer groups, some legislators, and even the fisheries themselves, *fish inspection is still not mandatory* at this writing for the more than 130,000 commercial fishing vessels and an estimated four thousand processing plants.[16]

When I first wrote *Poisons in Your Food* in 1969, there were eight hundred U.S. Food and Drug Administration inspectors for the more than 100,000 food, drug, and cosmetic plants in the United States. Today, there are fourteen hundred inspectors for about 102,000 food, animal drug, human drug, radiological, medical device, and cosmetic companies for which the FDA is responsible. The food manufacturing business alone is a six-hundred-billion-dollar-a-year industry, while the entire FDA yearly budget for food surveillance is only $132 million.[17]

The American Medical Association noted in 1989 that the FDA's effectiveness has been hampered by a 15 percent reduction in total personnel during the past decade, even while the agency's responsibilities have been significantly expanded by the passage of twenty-three new laws.[18]

When I first wrote *Poisons in Your Food,* our market shelves contained eight thousand items compared with the fifteen hundred they displayed before World War II. Today, the shelves are stocked with ten thousand items.

In 1987, the most recent year for which figures are available, ten thousand *new* grocery products were introduced to consumers, up about 25 percent over the seventy-five hundred new products in 1986.[19] But this constant increase in new items has created new dangers.

The technological changes that occur in processing certain foods can outstrip government and industry efforts to evaluate and control health hazards associated with new products and processes.

In 1971 I quoted Howard Bauman, Ph.D., then a vice-president of the Pillsbury Company, who, at the American Health Association–sponsored National Conference on Food Protection, warned of a "mass catastrophe" in the U.S. food supply. "Can you imagine the runways and control towers of the thirties trying to keep track of and land jets at our airports today? It seems ridiculous, but that's exactly what we're doing in the food business," Dr. Bauman said.[20]

Indeed, in 1985 the United States had the largest documented outbreak of foodborne illness in the nation's history. The cause was bacterial contamination in a *single* Illinois milk plant, contamination that affected approximately 200,000 people.[21]

An epidemiologist with the Centers for Disease Control in Atlanta, whose job it is to track the incidence of illnesses, admits that the reports of foodborne diseases that do filter in to the centers are only the tip of the iceberg and that the number of true outbreaks is actually fifty to one hundred times greater than the number reported.[22]

Since I first wrote this book, women have increasingly traded in the kitchen for the office. Food processors have responded to the need for a "fast preparation meal" that may literally be eaten on the run.

Microwave ovens exist to save time for the harried. In 1978, only 11 percent of American homes had them. Today, these quick-cooking devices are in 80 percent of our homes. The number of foods processed especially for microwaving is skyrocketing.

Spending on food to be consumed at home—food purchased mainly from supermarkets—has grown only by 20 percent since 1965, but spending on foods eaten away from home—at fast-food restaurants, delis, and other places that prepare food—has shot up by 89 percent, according to the United States Department of Agriculture.[23]

Those foods that are easier to prepare pass through many hands, to be mashed, mushed, mangled, and loaded with chemicals so that we can have instant cake mixes, instant potatoes, and instant everything else. You should remember that with every hand your food passes through and with each thing that is added to preserve and flavor it, the nutrition goes down and risk to your health goes up.

The use of chemicals in foods has soared from 419 million pounds in 1955 to more than 800 million today. Each of us eats more than fifty pounds of food additives a year, according to Robert Scheuplein, Ph.D., Office of Toxicological Sciences, Center for Food Safety, Food and Drug Administration.[24] Who tests these chemicals before they are added to our food? Who monitors their use and physical effects on use once they are in our diet?

In September 1980, the National Toxicology Program (NTP) contracted with the National Research Council (NRC) of the National Academy of Sciences for the NRC to determine the tests needed to truly evaluate the toxicity of common chemicals. The aim was to give to those government agencies responsible for protecting our health enough information to make a sound judgment.

The NRC considered 8,627 food additives in use.[25] For the great majority of the substances, the NRC found that data considered to be essential for evaluating a health hazard was either totally absent or lacking (see page 258). Therefore, it is not surprising that Linda Tollefson, Chief, Clinical Nutrition Assessment Section, U.S. Food and Drug Administration, points out, "We do not even know the true extent of adverse reactions to foods."[26]

But even if a food ingredient has definitely been proven to be a cancer-causing agent, it is more difficult today to remove it from our diet than it was twenty years ago, when the first edition of *Poisons in Your Food* was published.

The food industry has repeatedly attacked the Delaney Food Additives Amendment, public law 85-929, passed on December 6, 1958. The law specifically states that *no additive may be permitted in any amount if tests show that it produces cancer when fed to man or animals or by other appropriate tests.*

Ironically, the Delaney barrier began to weaken with the public's desire to keep the artificial sweetener saccharin on the market. Cyclamates, another artificial sweetener, had been removed from the store shelves earlier because tests indicated it might cause bladder tumors. Saccharin, in use since 1879, was then linked to cancer in animals. In 1977, the FDA announced that the use of saccharin in foods and beverages would be banned. There was a public outcry from dieters, led by the Calorie Control Council, a trade organization that spent over a million dollars in the first six months to stop the ban. Saccharin is still on the market, the FDA having postponed the ban several times in response to "public" pressure.

Since the first edition of this book appeared, the FDA has quietly adopted the *de minimis* approach to cancer-causing agents in the food supply. Such an interpretation is generally considered to mean that the law does not care for, or take notice of, trifling matters,[27] and allows the FDA to compare risk and benefit when issuing or revoking approval for an additive. But—a question asked throughout this book—whose risk and whose benefit? The FDA is breaking the law by ignoring the Delaney Amendment, and, unfortunately, when it comes to potentially harmful food additives, we take the risk while the food processor takes the benefits.[28]

The food industry has also been pushing for other changes in the food laws.[29] Among the new legislation they want:

- A definition of the term "safe," since a zero-risk standard is neither realistic nor desirable, they claim.
- Permission for a *gradual phaseout* of a product, since immediate bans on food additives disrupt the food supply and can cause severe economic hardship.

Want to know how *gradual* a phaseout can be? Take carbyl, a cancer-causing pesticide, for example. Rachel Carson, in her 1962 pioneering book *Silent Spring,* reported how fruit flies, the classic subject of genetics experiments, develop damaging and even fatal mutations when exposed to a group of chemicals called carbamates, from which many insecticides and other agricultural chemicals are drawn. Four years later, in its *Yearbook,* the United States Department of Agriculture noted that carbaryl, a carbamate, accumulates in human tissues.[30]

In 1989—twenty-seven years after Rachel Carson first sounded the alarm—the FDA said that carbyl should be removed from the market because it causes liver cancer. As of this writing, carbyl, aldicarb, and other carbamates are still being used and we are still getting residues in our food.

While the testing of additives in our food for induction of cancer may be imperfect, little if any testing is being done to determine if food additives may be toxic to the brain and nerves, although a number of scientists now believe that neurotoxins are even more of a problem in food than are cancer-causing agents.[31] (Read about the links between brain degeneration and pesticides in chapter 2, for example.)

Until relatively recently, scientists believed that the placenta protected the unborn child from toxic chemicals. The birth of children addicted to drugs because their mothers were addicted, and the recognition of fetal alcohol syndrome, in which babies are brain-damaged because their mothers drank liquor while pregnant, have proved the womb is not invulnerable to toxins. It is now evident that not only can chemicals penetrate the placenta and affect the unborn child, but that the chemicals may become more concentrated and more toxic. All children born in the United States today have traces of pesticides in their tissues.[32]

Concentration of a toxic agent in a child's body is especially hazardous. For example, infants and children may be at greater risk from the same level of a contaminant in water than are adults, according to Rita Meyninger, president of Environmental Systems Management and Design in Fort Lee, New Jersey.[33] In 1980, Meyninger was the chief federal official for the health emergency at Love Canal, where pollution of the ground and water by chemical contaminants from an industrial plant forced people to abandon their homes.

Meyninger explains that if, each day, a 22-pound child and a 154-pound adult both drink eight cups of water containing 1.7 milligrams per cup of a chemical, the child will receive a dosage three and a half times more damaging than that of the adult because of their difference in body size. In addition, Meyninger says, because children's gastrointestinal tracts more easily absorb nutrients than those of adults and because children absorb toxic agents more efficiently, a child will actually be at ten times greater risk than an adult from the same dose of chemical ingested.

Dr. James Watson, who won a Nobel Prize for his work in genetics, told me at a science writers' conference in New York in 1971: "Americans are very casual about what they do to their genes." He pointed out that we carelessly introduce chemicals into our environment without knowing their long-term effect.

One thing the food regulators and producers fail to take into consideration is that a minute residue of a harmful chemical in our diet is not isolated from other minute amounts of harmful chemicals in our medicines. Americans are the most medicated people in the world. Every year we swallow billions of doses of therapeutic pills, powders, capsules, and elixirs.

In addition to the foods we eat and the medicines we take, we fill the sky with 130 million tons of noxious chemicals . . . carbon monoxides, hydrocarbons, nitrogen oxides, sulfur oxides, and particulates. People living in New York City may inhale the equivalent of 730 pounds of chemicals a year.[34]

Our water today contains all sorts of pollutants, from detergents to sewage and industrial wastes.

The Clean Water Act may establish drinking-water standards based on the exposure of a healthy male adult who consumes eight cups of water per day. But there are other means of exposure to polluted water than swallowing it. Many chemicals in water may be inhaled after they have been made airborne in showers, dishwashers, and washing machines, or they may be absorbed through the skin during bathing, showering, or swimming. In fact, recent research has shown that the combination of inhaling chemicals into the lungs and absorbing them through the skin may contribute more to the total body burden of some toxins than does eating or drinking them.[35]

In addition to all the chemicals in food, water, medicine, and air, a large percentage of the population smokes and/or drinks alcoholic beverages. Tobacco smoke may be an additional cancer-causing agent that breaks down the body's immunity, while alcohol may be a solvent that aids another noxious chemical.

Industry and government scientists keep trying to reassure us by referring to "no-effect levels" and pointing out that one part per billion (ppb) of a substance in a food product is equal to one inch in sixteen thousand miles. But they never tell us how much exposure to a carcinogen it takes to damage a gene or to cause cancer in a child or adult, or what happens when you take in a combination of chemicals. No one knows!

The human body is a wondrous thing. It can detoxify many poisons through its liver and kidneys. It can fend off many germs and even cancer-causing agents—that is, if the body belongs to a young, healthy adult. But what about unborn children, infants, invalids, AIDS patients, and the elderly, whose resistance is not as great as that of a young healthy adult? What about those with damaged kidneys and livers? allergies? chronic illnesses?

Many eminent physicians, university scientists, politicians, and industrialists contend that the American food supply is wholesome, safe, and nutritious and that it is abundant. Compared with what the starving peoples of the world must eat, and in contrast with the typhoid- or tuberculosis-contaminated food of the past, perhaps we should not complain. It is true that our food is abundant to the point where our taxes pay farmers not to grow crops.

There is no doubt that food scientists, growers, processors, distributors, and sellers want to give us wholesome, appetizing foods. They want our dollars and our loyalty. The majority of city, state, and federal inspectors want to do a good job. They are consumers too.

But the job is too big, our desires too fickle, and the staffing and money too small to really protect us. Your best defense against contaminated, unhealthy food is your own knowledge and discrimination. *Not everything causes cancer. Not all foods are bad for you.* This book was written to report the current food hygiene situation and to help you make more informed and healthier choices.

2 ~ How to Kill Insects— and People

It was a warm June day—warm enough for a young mother to keep the window open while she gave her five-year-old son a bath. An insecticide that was being used to protect the elm trees in front of the house was accidentally whooshed through the window, filling the bathroom with fumes. Both the mother and the little boy choked and coughed for fifteen minutes.

Eight months later, the child was taken to the family physician because a skin wound had failed to heal properly. Worried about the slow healing and the boy's loss of appetite, listlessness, and enlarged spleen, the doctor had him admitted to the hospital for further tests. An examination of the child's blood marrow confirmed the dread diagnosis: acute granulocytic leukemia.

The child was treated by various means—the latest drugs, X rays, blood transfusions—but as spring was just beginning to fill the air and the elm trees in front of the house were once again proudly displaying their buds, the little boy died.

The following February his mother was referred to the Mayo Clinic because of a suspiciously low white blood count that had first been noticed three months earlier, when she suffered an attack of the flu with a fever of 103°. Her fever had cleared and she had felt well—that is, as well as a mother who has lost a child can ever feel.

At the hospital, an examination of her bone marrow revealed

acute leukemia. She was put on drugs and received twenty-eight blood transfusions. But, as did her little boy, she also succumbed to leukemia.[1]

High in the Andes of Colombia there is a town called Chiquinquirá, about which almost no one had heard until one November day. Chiquinquirá, like farm towns everywhere, rose early for breakfast that particular morning. By 8:30 A.M., the first child was dead. By afternoon, more than 130 persons, most of them children, violently sick and near death, had been brought to the hospital.

What was the deadly poison? About a pint of the pesticide parathion. On the hundred-mile truck journey from Bogotá, a parathion container had broken in its carton, and the insecticide leaked into the bags of flour. A baker used two of the bags of flour for his early morning batch of bread. Within four hours, the first of the victims had died.[2]

These two incidents of fatal pesticide poisoning involved relatively large doses. I noted in 1969 that "the awful question" haunting many scientists was whether the one to a dozen pesticides we may ingest with every meal might cause or contribute to a slow poisoning of our system and those of our unborn children. I also pointed out that little was known about the long-term effects of pesticides on children and the elderly, and that no one knew what happened when pesticides combine with each other or with the myriad chemicals in our environment. The American Academy of Pediatrics (AAP) in 1989 issued a fact sheet stating that the organization was forming a coalition with American Public Health Association to spur congressional action concerning environmental hazards. In the fact sheet the AAP pointed out: "Children are particularly sensitive to pesticides because their rapidly growing cells are more vulnerable to carcinogens than [are the cells of] adults " and that "over the lifetime of today's preschoolers, an estimated 4.5 million will contract cancer; approximately 5,000 of these cases may be caused by pesticides."[3]

In the 1970s, the Environmental Protection Agency (EPA) banned many of the "organochlorine" insecticides—DDT and its relatives—from general use because of public outcry over their residues in humans and wildlife. Yet the ecological and health effects of pesticides continue to plague us. The chemicals that have replaced the organochlorines—such as the organophosphates, including malathion and parathion (the culprit in the Colombian incident), and the carbamates such as carbaryl and aldicarb—are less persistent but they are also more water soluble and therefore more likely to reach living things in water and, eventually, us. Many of these materials are more instantly toxic, thus posing a greater hazard to farm workers in particular.

Since the first edition of *Poisons in Your Food,* information has been evolving from large studies of farmers exposed by occupation to agrichemicals over a period of time. The findings, thus far, are not reassuring.

FARMER'S HARVEST OF CANCER
Background

The impetus for the farming studies came from cancer atlases published in the mid-1970s that showed the geographic variations in many types of cancer deaths across the United States for the years 1950–1969. The atlases were published by the National Cancer Institute's Epidemiology and Biostatistics Program.

The color-coded maps revealed that death rates for blood and lymph cancers were elevated in rural regions in the central United States. A striking band indicating deaths from leukemia ran through counties in the central states from North Dakota to Texas. For non-Hodgkin's lymphoma (solid tumors of the lymph glands) and multiple myeloma (relatively rare bone-marrow cancer), rates were high in the north central states.

From the maps, NCI epidemiologists selected states to study where farming was a major occupation and death rates for blood and lymph cancers were above average. They found that the number of deaths from leukemia was elevated in areas where there was heavy production of corn, cotton, and wheat, and where pesticides were used.

Scientists at the National Cancer Institute conducted a series of nine studies over eight years to confirm that farmers, because of exposures in their work, were, indeed, at increased risk for some cancers.

DEATH CERTIFICATE STUDIES
Leukemia in Nebraska and Wisconsin

In a study of deaths from leukemia in Nebraska, the NCI epidemiologists found that farmers had a 25 percent greater risk of developing leukemia than did nonfarmers. The risk was greatest among farmers who were born after 1900 and died before the age of sixty-six—the age group that used the most pesticides. The NCI investigators also found high risk for leukemia in heavy corn-producing counties.

Another NCI study examined risk for leukemia among farmers in Wisconsin, where dairy farming is a major activity. It produced findings similar to those of the Nebraska study. The risk for developing leukemia was 10 percent greater for dairy farmers than it was for nonfarmers. The risk was again greatest among farmers who had the most exposure to chemical pesticides and among farmers from counties where chemical fertilizer was used heavily—as it was in the big corn-producing counties in Nebraska.[4]

For unknown reasons, chronic myeloid leukemia (a disease involving immature bone-marrow cells) occurred among the Wisconsin farmers 80 percent more frequently than did other cell-type leukemias. In the general adult population, chronic myeloid leukemia accounts for only 7 percent of leukemia deaths.

Non-Hodgkin's Lymphoma in Wisconsin

Dr. Kenneth Cantor investigated the risk to Wisconsin farmers of developing non-Hodgkin's lymphoma. Dr. Cantor found that Wisconsin farmers were almost twice as likely as nonfarmers to develop non-Hodgkin's lymphoma. The greatest risk was to those in the same age groups as those in the Nebraska and Wisconsin leukemia studies.[5]

"Of particular interest is the strength of the association seen between farming and risk for the cancer among farmers who died before the age of 66," he said. "This is noteworthy because the latency period after exposure to a carcinogen is generally believed to be about 20 years. This suggests that exposure to one or more agricultural chemicals first introduced in large volumes about 20 years before the time covered in the study—just after World War II—may be linked to the cancer."

The Wisconsin farmers were from counties with a high percentage of small grain acreage and acres treated with insecticides.

Multiple Myeloma in Wisconsin

Focusing on risk for multiple myeloma (a relatively rare bone-marrow cancer) among farmers, another study in Wisconsin indicated, again, that the rate was high among younger farmers who lived in areas where insecticides were heavily used.[6] Dr. Cantor also found that risk was increased for farmers who had lived in counties with a high percentage of chicken farming and fertilizer use.

These epidemiological studies suggested that agricultural practices could be linked to certain cancers, but in order to identify specific chemicals, the NCI researchers needed to question farmers directly.

INTERVIEW STUDIES
Non-Hodgkin's Lymphoma, Hodgkin's Disease, and Soft-tissue Sarcoma in Kansas

Farmers who had non-Hodgkin's lymphoma, Hodgkin's disease, and soft-tissue sarcoma were of interest because earlier studies had linked them with herbicide (weed killer) exposure, explained Dr. Sheila Hoar Zahm, who led the investigation.[7] (Herbicides are considered pesticides.) Kansas was selected because wheat is its major crop, and herbicides have been used on wheat more frequently than have other pesticides. Kansas was also chosen because it has a statewide tumor registry.

The Kansas farmers who used herbicides for more than twenty days each year risked developing non-Hodgkin's lymphoma six times more than nonfarmers did. Among these frequent users, those who mixed or applied the herbicides to the weeds themselves had eight times the risk. These above-normal rates were associated with the use of phenoxy herbicides, especially 2,4-D. Phenoxy herbicides are frequently used on pastureland and in growing wheat, corn, sorghum, and rice. The farmers who didn't use herbicides did not have the increased risk.

Leukemia and Non-Hodgkin's Lymphoma in Iowa and Minnesota

In Iowa and Minnesota analyses by cell type of the cancer suggested that risk for small-cell cancer of the lymph glands may be nearly one and a half times greater for farmers than for nonfarmers, particularly among farmers who used high volumes of pesticides twenty or more years ago. Risk for all types of non-Hodgkin's lymphoma appeared to be elevated among users of certain chlorinated hydrocarbon insecticides (such as DDT).

The epidemiologists found an increase in risk of nearly one and a half times for chronic lymphocytic leukemia associated with corn production. More farmers who had leukemia than those who did not had used dichlorvos on animals. (Dichlorvos is an insecticide and antiworm compound that inhibits cholinesterase, an enzyme important to nerve action. It is permitted in animal feed, and up to 0.1 part per million [ppm] is allowed by the FDA in edible tissues of swine. It is also in many household insecticides.) The Iowa and Minnesota farmers with the cancer also had more frequently used a group of pesticides that included DDT, methoxychlor, and nicotine.

Farmers, of course, have greater exposure to agricultural chemicals, but their cancers serve as an early warning to us. Accidental exposures to pesticides that result in acute ill-effects also portend chronic ill-effects over a period of time.

In *The Silent Spring,* Rachel Carson made the world aware of the potential dangers of pesticides. For an all-too-brief period, there was a great public outcry for stricter laws and controls. The reassuring books and articles flooded the market—most of them sponsored by pesticide manufacturers. Rachel Carson was accused of being a sensationalist, and the public settled back into apathy.

When Carson wrote *The Silent Spring,* farmers were using an estimated 175,826,000 pounds of five hundred different insecticidal chemicals. At the time of this writing, farmers are using more than a billion pounds—a tenfold increase since World War II—and more than thirteen hundred insecticidal chemicals.[8]

In 1969, I quoted Agricultural Research Division entomologist C. H. Hoffman and chief of the Stored Product Insect Research Branch L. S. Henderson, both of the United States Department of Agriculture: "Without insecticides, production of livestock would soon drop about 25 percent and production of crops about 30 percent. Food prices might then go up as much as 50 to 75 percent and the food still not be of high quality."[9]

Yet, more than twenty years later, Michael Dover, writing in *Technology Review,* pointed out: "Heavy reliance on synthetic pesticides has also spawned problems that jeopardize effective pest control itself. For example, many species of pests are becoming immune to the effects of these chemicals. From 1970 to 1980 the number of such resistant species of arthropods—insects, mites, and ticks—jumped from 224 to 428. The numbers of resistant species of rodents' bacteria, fungi and weeds are also increasing. Resistance threatens the future of potato farming in the Northeastern United States and cotton growing in several parts of the world. In the tropics, resistance also impedes control of insect-borne diseases: the chemical industry can no longer develop new pesticides as quickly as pests develop immunity."[10]

Farmers must pay more and more for less and less effective chemicals. We are paying more for our food. The real question is whether the price farmers and the rest of us are paying for pesticides may be cancer, birth defects, liver diseases, and even mental illness.

Farmers, at least, use pesticides deliberately. We swallow them unintentionally.

BOOBY-TRAPPED WATERMELON

Take aldicarb, for example. It has long been a worry because it is so poisonous. One drop absorbed through the skin can kill an adult. Farmers apply it in granules to reduce risk.

As a summer tradition, many celebrants in California and Oregon ate watermelon on July 4, 1985, as they had picnics and watched fireworks. Within hours, hundreds of those who had consumed watermelon become violently ill, developing symptoms ranging from nausea and diarrhea to seizures, blurred vision, and irregular heartbeat. Belatedly, the Food and Drug Administration discovered that a large number of California watermelons were contaminated with aldicarb.[11]

Reports of illness associated with eating watermelons continued to pour in through most of July, bringing the total to 1,350. When laboratory analyses were run on the contaminated melons, it was found that, in many cases, residue levels that had made people sick were well below those that the FDA's routine screening tests can detect.

For officials at both the FDA and the Environmental Protection Agency, the most worrisome aspect of the contamination outbreak was the question of how aldicarb ever got into watermelons in the first place. An insecticide primarily used to treat citrus and potato crops, aldicarb cannot legally be used on melons. One theory held that the melons had absorbed the chemical from tainted groundwater, which can remain contaminated with the pesticide for years. The explanation turned out to be that three California watermelon growers had illegally used aldicarb on their crops.

In New York, ten years before the western watermelon fiasco, New York authorities investigating mysterious stomach ailments in Suffolk County, Long Island, found the amount of aldicarb in underground water to be fifty times higher than that considered safe by the EPA. It was being used on potato crops.

What's the story on aldicarb today?

On January 12, 1989—four years after the booby-trapped watermelon incident and fourteen years after the Long Islanders' bout with pesticide-contaminated water—Environmental Protection Agency toxicologists recommended that the use of aldicarb be restricted on bananas and potatoes because of the danger to the health of infants and children exposed to its residues. The report said that each day fifteen thousand to fifty thousand infants and children are exposed to enough aldicarb from eating potatoes to be at risk of getting ill. Bananas were said to present a risk to as many as fifteen hundred infants and children.[12]

The use of aldicarb on ten other crops, however, is still allowed to continue under the recommendations because the chemical is not used as heavily as it is on potatoes and bananas, and the residues are not as high.

The farmers and the cases of accidental poisonings mentioned so far concern relatively large doses of pesticides. The government agencies, many university experts, and manufacturers of agriculture chemicals assure us that we are exposed to only harmless, minute amounts of pesticide residues. Just a brief look at the scientific literature used for this book shows that such assurance is not based on fact but on wishful thinking.

First of all, pesticides in air, water, and earth travel hundreds of thousands of miles from the place they are first used, as numerous reports have shown. They may also persist for years in the soil, either in their original form or in broken-down products. Nor is there any known way in which the drift of agricultural chemicals can be entirely eliminated, whether such attempts are made on the ground or from aircraft. If pesticides are sprayed by plane, 50 percent of the chemical is lost to drift. How far the pesticide drifts depends on the size of the droplets and the speed of the wind. Drift of tracers used in air pollution studies has been authenticated as far as twenty-two miles and greater distances are possible depending on the accuracy of the means for sensing tracer chemicals.[13]

DANGEROUS FOG

Researchers at USDA research laboratories in Beltsville, Maryland, reported at an American Chemical Society meeting in 1989 that they had developed a method of analyzing the content of fog samples.[14]

They collected fog and air samples along the Pacific Coast near Monterey, California, and inland to the Coast Ranges. Samples taken near the coast were in vegetable-crop-growing areas, while the samples taken farther inland were in largely nonagricultural areas. Diazon, methyl parathion, malathion, methidathion, chlorpyrifos, carbaryl, dyfonate, and breakdown products of the parent pesticides were found in what was expected to be relatively clean coastal fog.[15]

WHAT'S IN THE WATER

Some of the pesticide sprayed from the air winds up in the waters of lakes. A persistent pesticide introduced into a body of water may concentrate in different parts of the food chain. An instance of such "biological magnification" can be seen in waters that contain 0.02 ppm of a persistent pesticide while producing plankton containing 5 ppm and fish containing hundreds of thousands of parts per million. Then we eat the fish and get an even higher dose of pesticides. Moreover, fields sprayed with pesticides have plants as well as bugs that absorb the chemical, which may again lead to "biological magnification."

Take the case of the pesticide heptachlor, which accumulates in animal and milk fats and has been found to be especially dangerous for nursing mothers, infants, and children. In animal studies, heptachlor causes malignant tumors. In what was to become known as the fire-ant fiasco, a million acres of southern land were dusted with a concoction of heptachlor formulated to remain effective in soil for at least three years. It was aimed at killing the red ants that bite and cause damage to people and crops. This program continued for more than a year before it was discovered that weathering in soil transforms heptachlor into the very persistent and poisonous epoxide.[16]

Almost every use of the chemical was outlawed after the fire-ant fiasco in 1978—many years after it had been sprayed on crops and residues were in our foods.

But heptachlor has not disappeared!

WHAT'S IN ANIMAL FEED

One of the nation's largest poultry producers destroyed four hundred thousand chickens in 1989 because the birds were contaminated with heptachlor. Although the pesticide was banned for use in food eleven years before, the Environmental Protection Agency has continued to allow farmers and feed companies to use existing supplies on corn, wheat, sorghum, barley, oat, and rye seeds to protect them against insects.

The EPA estimates that sixty thousand to eighty thousand gallons of heptachlor are still available for treating grain seeds, enough to last eighty years. Moreover, a virtually unregulated trade has developed for grain seeds treated with toxic pesticides like heptachlor that are outlawed for use in food. The chemicals are used on seeds to prevent damage before planting and during germination.

The destruction of the chickens was the most serious known incident of pesticide contamination in the history of Arkansas's three-billion-dollar poultry industry, the largest in the nation. But it was the fourth time since 1981 that food products in the state had been contaminated with toxic insecticides outlawed in the 1970s. Two of those incidents involved poultry and two contaminated milk. Similar incidents have occurred in dairy cows in Hawaii and dairy cows and pigs in Indiana.[17]

Investigators believe the Arkansas chicken fiasco was caused by sorghum seeds sprayed and sold illegally for feed. When the government allowed existing stocks of heptachlor to be used, it directed that treated seeds be dyed red as a warning to livestock and poultry producers. Sorghum seeds are rust-colored, so the red-dye "warning" could easily have been missed. The seeds were purchased by the Townsend Poultry Products plant in Arkansas and mixed into feed that was distributed to many of the 196 farmers who raise chickens for the company under contract.

The contamination was discovered on January 4, 1989, in tests conducted, not by government agents, but by Campbell Soup Company personnel in Fayetteville. Campbell's had purchased two hundred pounds of meat from Townsend to use in experimenal runs for a new product. The Campbell soup plant processes chickens into parts for Swanson brand frozen dinners and is one of the food companies in Arkansas that routinely monitors feed and chickens for residues of about three hundred pesticides.

Campbell's tests showed that the levels of heptachlor discovered in Townsend meat ranged to 2.4 ppm. The level considered safe by federal health authorities is 0.3 ppm.

To prevent another costly disaster, Townsend has instituted procedures to more thoroughly test all the grain it uses in chicken feed and to conduct residue tests of chickens days before they are slaughtered. But what if Campbell's personnel in Fayetteville hadn't checked those chickens? Would Townsend now be testing feed? Would those chickens have reached our tables?

Heptachlor showed up before, in milk. In 1983, much of Hawaii's milk supply was found to be contaminated by heptachlor. Nor is heptachlor the only pesticide residue that is cause for alarm. In 1984, the nation's grain supply, citrus crops, and other foods were found to contain the powerful chemical ethylene dibromide, which causes cancer and birth defects. In 1988 and 1989, consumers learned that some supplies of apple juice might have been tainted with a "growth regulator," Alar (daminozide), which was previously linked to cancer in tests conducted by the National Cancer Institute.[18]

The list could go on and on. In fact, the National Academy of Sciences, a semigovernment agency, released a study in 1987 that concluded that ten pesticides that are known to cause cancer and that have been found in foods might cause more than one million cancers over the next seventy years.[19]

What percentage of pesticide-contaminated products reaches our plates without anyone ever knowing? Are we being harmed over a period of time by agricultural chemical residues in our food, air, and water?

PHYSICAL EFFECTS OF PESTICIDES

Detecting the physical effects of pesticide residues is difficult to do unless there is an acute and dramatic widespread illness due to pesticides, such as happened during the watermelon incident on the West Coast and the Long Island potato incident. Symptoms of slow, low-dose poisoning may go undiagnosed; there are even cases of large-dose poisonings that are unrecognized.

Dr. Irma West, of the Bureau of Occupational Health, State of California Department of Public Health, said before a Senate committee in 1963: "With the notable exception of the organic phosphate pesticides, physicians do not have laboratory tests available to confirm diagnoses of agricultural chemical poisoning. Diagnoses can be made on a clinical or circumstantial basis only. Signs and symptoms may be similar to many other conditions. Just about any illness can be attributed to chemicals and there is little help in confirming, refuting for clarifying the situation. Bona fide cases can be buried among the erroneous, and vice versa.

"There are instances of the most astute diagnostic skill and examples of the most dismal ignorance in the medical handling of pesticide poisoning."[20]

As an example of the latter, she cited the case of a young boy who had been applying an organic phosphate pesticide all day and developed symptoms of poisoning. He was sent home twice over the course of several hours by the same physician. The first time the doctor sent the boy home with a tranquilizer.

"The second time the boy came for medical help," Dr. West said, "the label from the chemical was presented to the physician, who sent him home again with several atropine pills, a first aid recommendation on some labels but an entirely inadequate treatment. The boy died during the night at home, still in his contaminated work clothes."

A San Francisco psychiatrist, Dr. Douglas Gordon Campbell, of the University of California Medical School, was quoted in the first edition of this book: "Every physician should ask if the patient uses pesticide sprays in the home, in the garden, or on the job. Patients with obscure and seemingly neurotic symptoms are sometimes victims of chronic poisoning by such household sprays."[21]

He told of a patient who went from doctor to doctor, none of whom could diagnose his loss of coordination, blurred speech, and other neurological symptoms. A check of fatty tissue from the patient showed it contained six times the average amount of pesticide.

CHILDREN AND PESTICIDES

The Natural Resources Defense Council—a nonprofit environmentalist group—stirred up a furor in 1989 when it asked a new question about an old problem: What happens to allowable traces of those chemicals in our food that are set for a grownup but a child may not tolerate?[22]

The NRDC looked at a United States Department of Agriculture survey of the fruits and vegetables that American children eat. They used Food and Drug Administration data regarding the amounts of pesticide residues that are found in those foods. Then based on animal and in-vitro tests by the EPA, they added up the risks to young children.

The principal findings:

- The average preschooler has 400 percent greater total exposure than does an adult to the eight carcinogenic pesticides analyzed in the survey.
- A person typically receives 55 percent of the risk, over a lifetime of exposure, in the first five years.
- As a result of exposure during the early years, one child out of thirty-four hundred may develop cancer during his or her life.
- Up to half of all preschoolers may be exposed to unsafe levels of organophosphates (pesticides that kill insects by attacking their nervous system). Little children, with their nervous systems still developing, may be at special risk for nerve or brain damage, behavior disorders, or learning disabilities.

Two years before the NRDC report, Richard Jackson, M.D., formed chairman of the committee on environmental hazards of the American Academy of Pediatrics, said: "Of all the chemical hazards the public faces from polluted air, water, and food, pesticides in food pose the greatest risk."[23]

If children are at risk with their immature immune systems, so are the elderly with their failing immune systems.

In the first edition of this book, a Florida study of pesticide concentrations in fat tissue taken at human autopsies sounded an alarm. Drs. William B. Deichmann, J. L. Radomski, and Alberto Rey, all of the department of pharmacology and the Research and Teaching Center of Toxicology at the University of Miami Medical School, found that twice the amount of DDT, DDE, DDD, and dieldrin were in the fat of patients who died of liver or central nervous disease than appeared in the fat of those who died accidental deaths.[24]

In one case of amyloidosis (abnormal deposits of protein in organs or tissues), the Miami researchers found all pesticide levels were extremely high—the highest encountered.

This study, reported in 1968, has probably been lost under the weight of thousands of research papers that have come out every week since then on all sorts of topics. But to those with an interest in Alzheimer's disease, a devastating form of incurable and progressive brain degeneration that increasingly affects people over the age of sixty, it should be of interest. On being autopsied, the brains of Alzheimer's victims show not only aluminum deposits (see page 189) but severe amyloidosis.

In other studies included in the first edition of this book, researchers in Australia and at the University of Chicago found that organophosphates such as malathion and parathion irreversibly inhibit cholinesterase after lengthy exposure.[25] Cholinesterase is an enzyme in the brain, one needed to process acetylcholine, the chemical that carries messages between nerve cells and is vital to memory function. One of the factors in Alzheimer's and other memory problems of aging is that the acetylcholine signals between nerves are not working right.

The 1960s research also reported that prolonged exposure to organophosphorus insecticides may cause depressive or schizophrenic reactions, with impairment of memory and of concentration, two symptoms of Alzheimer's. Measurements of brain waves showed a slowed activity.

In still another possible connection between pesticides and the brain, André Barbeau, of the Clinical Research Institute in Montreal, collected data on the incidence of Parkinson's disease in the nine water regions of Quebec Province and matched them with pesticide use. The Montreal team used four independent methods to track the disease incidence and came up with more than five thousand cases. The correlation between disease incidence and level of pesticide use was very strong. An area southwest of Montreal, Quebec's breadbasket, recorded the highest rural incidence, 0.89 per thousand of population, compared with 0.13 per thousand in regions where pesticide use was low.[26]

One of the pesticides suspected of contributing to Parkinsonism is paraquat. The United States Food and Drug Administration permits paraquat residues ranging between three and six ppm on sunflower seeds and hulls and in mint hay. The FDA does not list an available test to monitor paraquat residues.[27]

Are the connections between pesticides and brain degeneration just a coincidence? Someone ought to find out.

Even when researchers do make correlations between long-term use and human peril, it may not cause the pesticide to be removed from the market or from your food.

Take the case of Captan, used for more than seventeen years to protect seeds against fungus that rots them. Measured by ordinary toxic effects, Captan is mild. The Food and Drug Administration regulations allow a residue of 100 ppm to be left on raw agricultural products, a limit set in 1958 after experiments with dogs, cattle, and poultry showed no toxic effects from much higher concentrations. In contrast, the residue limit for an insecticide such as chlordane is three-tenths of a part per million.

But in 1967, an FDA researcher discovered that Captan has disastrous effects on reproduction of cells. Structurally, it is similar to Thalidomide, which caused thousands of babies in Europe to be born without arms and legs.[28] According to the experiments of Dr. Marvin Legator of FDA's Cell Biology Research Branch, the chemical inhibits the production of DNA, the basic genetic stuff of life, and breaks up cell chromosomes. Dr. Legator, reporting to a symposium in Washington in 1967, said, "Captan is only one of a number of chemicals formerly considered safe that are now suspected of causing genetic damage."[29]

Not only can Captan cause birth defects, it is also a cancer-causing agent in animals.

The FDA still permits up to 50 ppm of Captan as a residue in or on washed raisins and 100 ppm on cornseed. An estimated 344,0000 pounds of Captan are used each year on table grapes, and residue of this compound is the most frequently discovered material on grapes in grocery stores.

WHO'S DOWN ON THE FARM AND IN THE MARKET?

The Environmental Protection Agency, the United States Department of Agriculture, and the Food and Drug Administration have joint responsibility in the area of pesticides.

The EPA registers or approves the use of pesticides and establishes tolerances if use of a pesticide may lead to residues in food. A "tolerance" is the maximum amount of a residue expected in a food when a pesticide chemical is used according to the label directions, provided that the level does not present an unacceptable health risk. In 1987, there were 320 pesticide chemicals with established food and/or feed tolerances in the United States.[30]

With the exception of meat and poultry, for which the USDA is responsible, the FDA is charged with enforcing tolerances on food shipped in interstate commerce and as part of these activities determines the incidence and levels of pesticide residues in domestically produced and imported foods.[31]

At the federal level, pesticides are currently regulated under the authority of the Federal Insecticide, Fungicide and Rodenticide Act of 1988 (FIFRA). There are two major problems with FIFRA.

The first is that FIFRA relies almost entirely on labeling to control the use of pesticides, and though many pesticide users fail to read the labels (they may not even be able to read English), and though many who do read them ignore the instructions that they contain, this is really the only control we have.

At the twelfth annual national migrant-health conference in Indianapolis in 1989, Cesar Chavez, founder and president of the United Farm Workers of America, said: "While growers and foremen tell the unsophisticated workers that pesticides are 'harmless medicine for the plants,' and the EPA maintains that 'a little poison won't hurt you,' the actual result of exposure to them [pesticides] may be cancer, severe nerve disorders, reproductive problems, including teratogenicity [causing birth defects] and infertility, liver and kidney disease, and other illnesses." He is campaigning to end the use of these pesticides in this country.[32]

In 1989, George Hamilton, Ph.D., pesticide coordinator, Rutgers University Cooperative Extension Service, Cook College, said during a lecture at Kings Supermarket in Short Hills, New Jersey, that "everything FIFRA says must be done shows up on the product label—directions for use, safety, or hazards to humans and the environment."

I asked him, "If workers are illegal immigrants and/or illiterate, how can they read the label?"

He said, "Depending on the type of the material, there is a certification program in New Jersey and only certain persons can use 'restricted' pesticides. You have to take exams in English to be certified. If they can't read the label, they shouldn't be applying it. Basically, you won't be able to buy 'restricted' pesticides unless you are under somebody's supervision that does have a license."

"How do you police it?" I asked.

"Basically, the department has a division of pesticide control, and they have an enforcement section within that division and their inspectors go to farms and landscape firms. They check the records of applications and they do a lot of responding to complaints from the public, from organizations . . . from anywhere."

"How many inspectors?" I asked. "And how much territory do they have to cover?"

Professor Hamilton said, "Ten inspectors and they must cover farms, landscapers, commercial applicators . . . at least ten thousand locales."

He said most state departments have similar setups, although not all require pesticide applicators to be certified.

"What's the punishment," I asked, "if one of the state health department inspectors should catch someone—certified or not—applying pesticides incorrectly?"

In New Jersey, he said, there is a fee schedule for violations, ranging anywhere from fifty dollars to a maximum of three thousand dollars per violation. Violation of a tolerance level of pesticides in a material can result in confiscation of the crop, which, he said, is a greater hardship than is a three-thousand-dollar fine.

The second major problem with FIFRA is that the procedures for registration, cancellation, and suspension of pesticides are either inadequate or are very cumbersome. Often several years pass between the time a cancellation order is issued and the time that it becomes effective.

CHANGE IN FIFRA LAW

The amendments to the Federal Insecticide, Fungicide and Rodenticide Act were signed into law on October 25, 1988. This represents the first major change to the federal pesticide law since 1978. The act specifies that the EPA must issue regulations for the design of safe pesticide containers and promote the safe storage and disposal of pesticides no later than December 1991.

More than thirteen hundred chemicals were used as active ingredients in pesticide products registered before November 1984, but many have been dropped in response to requirements for new data and study standards to support continued registration.

The Environmental Protection Agency estimated that about 600 active pesticide ingredients would be reviewed under reregistration provisions of the 1988 amendments to FIFRA. About 70 of the 600 ingredients, however, were voluntarily taken off the market because of new data about their dangers.

Companies already registered to produce pesticides have been asked whether they intend to seek reregistration, and if so, what existing data and new studies they are going to use to assure the safety of their products.[33]

MORE CHANGES IN FIFRA NEEDED

In 1989, the Environmental Protection Agency reacted to growing public concern that the government regulation of agricultural chemicals was failing to keep dangerous substances out of the environment and the food supply.[34]

William K. Reilly, administrator of the EPA, presented a draft of the legislative proposal that said further changes were needed in the Federal Insecticide, Fungicide and Rodenticide Act to avoid the alarm over Alar (daminozide) and other farm chemicals.

The EPA first proposed banning Alar in 1985.

(Uniroyal Chemical Co., bowing to concerns about the safety of its controversial apple growth regulator, took it off the market June 3, 1989. As of this writing, you can still ingest Alar as a result of drinking apple juice made from concentrates imported from Europe and Argentina, which have more than a 50 percent share of the United States apple market.)

Today, the planned changes in FIFRA, which would need congressional approval, would streamline efforts to cancel the use of chemicals suspected of causing cancer or other disease by removing a judicial appeals process that chemical companies can now use to delay action. The process typically lasts four to eight years. Under the new system, the chemicals could be removed in two to four years. The proposal would also narrow the definition of economic benefits that can be used to justify allowing potentially dangerous chemicals to remain on the market.

The draft of the legislative proposal noted: "The Alar case illustrates that allowing continued use of pesticide products for years after significant health risks are indemnified results in loss of public confidence in Government's ability to protect their health."

The document said that Alar was not an isolated case and that as the agency examined more evidence about pesticides that have been on the market for many years, it would inevitably find some that presented high health risks.

The agency is also proposing that it be allowed to pull a chemical from the market while it is still investigating its potential risks; the current provision for an emergency suspension requires that there be relatively conclusive evidence of serious threat to public health.

Another major proposed change would affect the permissible residues of agricultural chemicals on food products. Residues are permitted if they represent a "negligible risk" to human health, but the rules allow consideration of other factors, particularly the benefits of the chemical to growers and to society as a whole. Under the proposed change only two benefits could be considered when determining if residues posing more than a negligible health risk will be permitted:

1. The health risks of the food would be higher than they would be without the use of the chemicals.

2. Absence of the pesticide would cause significant disruptions of the United States food supply, affecting availability of foods to lower income people or a massive shift to foreign sources of the food item.

WHO IS MONITORING RESIDUES?

Monitoring of pesticides is shared between the Food and Drug Administration and the United States Department of Agriculture.

In the first edition of *Poisons in Your Food,* I noted that the General Accounting Office (GAO), a congressional watchdog agency, accused the Agriculture Department of not acting aggressively enough to protect the public from "misbranded, adulterated, or unregistered" pesticides in a report sent to Congress in September 1968.

The 1968 report stated that the division had not taken action to prosecute violators of the pesticides control law to obtain recall of misbranded, adulterated, and unregistered products. Moreover, the agency found the division did not even obtain sufficient data to track defective products to different locations in the country.

There has not been much change since then. In fact, shortages of personnel and money may have made the situation worse. A corps of fourteen hundred FNA inspectors throughout the country are supposed to test for pesticides on domestic and imported foods. The FDA has concluded that it cannot monitor all food that may contain illegal pesticide residues. Consequently, it spot-checks a very small amount—*less than 1 percent of domestically produced food.*[35]

Since the FDA is short of manpower and money, it uses "selective surveys" to obtain information on specific pesticides and commodities and on a combination of pesticide, commodity, and country.[36]

An example of the first type of selective survey was carried out in 1987 for EBDCs (Ethylene-bisdithiocarbamate), a group of fungicides that are known to cause cancer in animals. Sixty-one samples representing ten different foods were analyzed. Thirty samples contained EBDC residues within legal limits. Three spinach samples, all from the same grower, contained EBDC residues that were in violation. The grower was advised of the FDA's findings and voluntarily destroyed twenty-five cases of harvested spinach and the unharvested spinach in two fields.[37] On December 4, 1989, the Environmental Protection Agency called for curbs on EBDC, saying widespread use of the chemical on scores of crops from apples to tomatoes poses an unreasonable cancer risk.[38]

An example of the second type of "selective survey" involved bananas. Eighty-eight banana samples, representing five countries, were analyzed. One or more residues were found in forty samples. Residues of five different pesticides were found, all at legal levels— that is, the residues were lower than the tolerance levels. As a result of such "selective surveys," or spot-checking, the FDA concluded that only 1.5 percent of the domestic and 3.4 percent of the import surveillance samples were in violation.

In addition to spot-checking using its own personnel, the FDA works with state authorities to develop cooperative sampling plans and information exchanges. The agency believes that this will result in more effective coverage of the domestic food supply and improve follow-up procedures to correct residue problems.

The FDA also has a contract with states to compile data on pesticides and industrial contamination of foods analyzed by state laboratories. The system, called Foodcon, contains results from about fifteen thousand samples received in 1987 from five states. A similar system, called Feedcon, is in place for animal feed data from the same five states.

The other major approach to pesticide monitoring used by the FDA is the Total Diet Study. Also known as the Market Basket Study, this effort is designed to estimate the dietary intake of pesticide residues by eight age-sex groups, from infants to senior citizens. (Industrial chemicals, heavy metals, radionuclides, and essential minerals are also measured.)

FDA personnel purchase foods from local supermarkets or grocery stores, just as you would, four times per year throughout the United States. Each of the four market basket samples is a composite of foods collected in three cities in a particular region. The cities of collection are changed each year. Each market basket contains 234 individual food items that have been chosen, based on nationwide dietary surveys, to represent the diet of the U.S. population. The foods are prepared table-ready (peeled, cooked, et cetera) and then are analyzed for pesticide residues. The results of these analyses, coupled with data on the amounts of these foods consumed, allow for calculations to be made of the dietary intakes of these residues. These provide estimates of the actual amount of pesticides consumed in foods as they are usually eaten.

The FDA determined that of the 200 chemicals that can be

detected by its laboratory procedures—there are no tests for many pesticides—53 pesticides were found in the 1987 market basket foods. The 27 pesticides most frequently found included:

- Malathion (23 percent of the time).
- DDT (22 percent of the time; restricted in use since the 1970s in the United States).
- Diazinon (21 percent of the time).
- Dieldrin (12 percent of the time).
- Hexachlorobenzene (10 percent of the time).

Among those foods found by the FDA in domestic sampling to be in violation were:

wheat	food sweeteners
Chinese cabbage	fruit
okra	dandelion greens
kale	parsley
spices	flavorings

The 1987 FDA summary of 14,492 samples of domestically produced and imported foods analyzed for pesticide residues from seventy-nine countries stated that no residues were found in 50 percent of the samples—but that means 50 percent of the samples did have pesticide residues. Most residues, according to the FDA, were at low levels and rarely exceeded tolerances. Less than 1 percent of the 14,492 samples contained residues that exceeded regulatory limits.

The FDA report for the latest findings states: "While the analytical methods used in the total diet study are capable of determining only about half the pesticides with United States' food tolerance, there is no compelling reason to believe that the situation regarding residue levels and corresponding intakes would be any different for those not detectable."

How are "safe" residue levels set?

The Acceptable Daily Intake (ADI) for dietary pesticides is established by the United Nations Food and Agriculture Organization and the World Health Organization as well as by the FDA market basket studies. An ADI is the daily intake of a chemical that, if ingested over a lifetime, appears to be without appreciable risk. For almost all pesticides the dietary intake is less than 1 percent of the ADI. Total Diet Study analyses focus on table-ready foods rather than on raw, unwashed, agricultural commodities because food preparation often reduces the levels of pesticide residues.

Just a note to remind those who set the ADI levels: In the West Coast watermelon outbreak of illness, actual laboratory studies of the contaminated watermelon and the blood of the patients showed that the residue levels of aldicarb in the watermelon that caused illness were often far below the level at which FDA screening tests can detect aldicarb.

The FDA pesticide domestic monitoring program as it is currently carried out has four major shortcomings.

1. The FDA does not regularly test food for a large number of pesticides that can be used or may be present in food. Included among these are a number of pesticides that, according to the FDA, require continuous or periodic monitoring because they are known as potential health hazards.

2. The FDA does not prevent the marketing of most of the food found during inspection to contain illegal pesticide residues.

3. The FDA does not penalize growers who market food with illegal pesticide residues when the agency is unable to remove it from the market.

4. Penalties are not being assessed for marketing adulterated food.

IMPORTED FOOD

The FDA is also responsible for checking imported foods for pesticides, and as it does with domestic foods, it "spot-checks." In one year, for example, only fourteen samples of oranges were taken out of the two billion pounds of oranges imported to this country. This is equivalent to one sample for every two hundred million pounds of imported oranges.[39]

Since the first edition of *Poisons in Your Food* appeared, many American farms have given way to housing developments, malls, and industrial parks. Our nation, which once led the world in abundance of farm produce, now imports larger and larger amounts of foreign products.

In 1986, the United States purchased a record $24.1 billion of imported food, a 40 percent rise from 1982. Fruit and vegetable imports led the increase, driven by United States consumer demand for fresh produce year-round. Fresh-fruit imports reached $1.2 billion in 1988, more than double the amount of 1979.[40]

Why should we worry about imported foods and pesticides?

United States pesticide makers are selling their banned products to foreign countries. Furthermore, poorly trained Third World farmers often use United States–approved pesticides at the wrong time, on the wrong crops, or in excessive amounts. In addition, Mexico, a major U.S. food supplier, has a poor safety record handling pesticides.[41]

In the last year alone, a number of pesticides banned by United States officials as public health threats have been found on imported produce. The compounds are suspected of producing cancer, neurological problems, and other ills. More commonly, the pesticides found on foreign produce are legal but exceed our approved levels or were sprayed on crops for which the United States hasn't approved their use.[42]

The FDA does not even test imported food items for the U.S. banned pesticide DBCP, a carcinogen known to cause sterility in males. Yet DBCP is reportedly used extensively worldwide, particularly on bananas and pineapples.

The U.S. General Accounting Office reported in September 1986 that the FDA's general sample selection criteria for imported food was high volume, dietary significance, and past pesticide problems.

The GAO found that between 1979 and 1985, the FDA collected and analyzed 33,687 imported food samples and discovered that 2,056 (6.1 percent) contained illegal residues. In addition, many foods imported from many countries are not being sampled. For example, shipments from only nine of twenty-seven countries exporting cucumbers to the United States from 1983 through 1985 have been sampled. The country exporting the second largest volume of cucumbers to the United States as well as sixteen other countries have not had their cucumber shipments sampled since at least 1978.

Among the foreign samples that were tested and found to have high residues were:

grain products
meats
grapes
peas
parsley
sweet potatoes

strawberries
other berries
black-eyed peas
corn
some vegetable oil products

Of the 164 adulterated samples that the GAO reviewed, 73 were not detained and were probably consumed by the public.

Federal agents who watch United States borders say that 6.1 percent of all food imports tested violate United States safety laws, double the rate for domestic produce. Yet a mere 1 percent of the estimated one million food shipments entering the United States annually are checked for dangerous pesticide residues, according to the September 1986 study by the General Accounting Office.

Before the FDA found cyanide in two Chilean grapes in 1989 and held up the import of the fruit until further tests could be done, most people did not know that the grapes on their tables came from Chile. Chileans knew it because fruit represents about 10 percent of Chile's total exports.

Mexico now supplies more than half the vegetables eaten by Americans. Mexican bell peppers were found, when tested, to be coated with benzene hexachloride, a suspected cancer-causing pesticide banned by United States regulators.

At the major United States border crossing for Mexican exports in Nogales, Arizona, food may enter the United States every weekday evening and throughout Friday and Saturday without pesticide checks. The reason: FDA pesticide inspectors aren't on duty. Even when the FDA does test the produce, its slow procedures prevent it from stopping 45 percent of the pesticide-tainted shipments headed for U.S. consumers, the GAO study found.

Importers handling tainted food need little fear punishment. Between 1979 and 1985, according to the GAO, the FDA levied fines in only 15 percent of the cases in which importers repeatedly violated United States food safety standards. Some 75 percent of those fines hadn't been collected by the FDA more than a year later.

The GAO has documented only eight cases where importers were assessed (for monetary damages). Damages in six of these cases had not even been collected a year after being assessed. This means that about 45 percent of the adulterated shipments are reaching consumers with few importers paying damages.

Politics play a part. Ethylene dibromide (EDB) was used for forty to fifty years as a gasoline additive; as a soil fumigant for worm control; as a means of protecting stored wheat, corn, and other grains against destruction by insects and contamination by molds and fungi; as a treatment for fruits against the spread of fruit flies; and as a tool to keep milling machinery free of insects. It was suspended in 1983 by the EPA because an "imminent hazard" to humans existed from groundwater contamination resulting from the use of EDB as a soil fumigant. But the agency allowed foreign mango growers to continue using the pesticide until 1985 while they tried to find alternatives. The pesticide, which is used abroad to kill fruit flies, penetrates the mangoes' skin and contaminates the flesh of the fruit.[43]

A foreign ban would have affected 80 percent of the mangoes eaten by United States consumers. State Department officials argued that a ban might be economically harmful to Mexico and Haiti, two major mango-exporting nations, as well as damaging to U.S.-financed mango-growing projects that relied on EDB in Belize and Guatemala.

The appeals court revealed that the EPA's failure to enforce the EDB ban placed "foreign well-being above the interest of U.S. consumers."

The GAO recommended that the secretary of the Department of Health and Human Services direct the FDA commissioner to:

- Redirect sampling coverage to a wider range of imported foods and countries.
- Consider several options for obtaining additional information on pesticides actually used in foreign food production and to test for these pesticides.

To select the proper test, the FDA should have information about pesticides actually used on foods produced in foreign countries.

Little such information is currently available. The GAO says that this problem could be solved if:

1. U.S. manufacturers who export pesticides to countries that export food to the United States had to inform the FDA of what they have sold.

2. Importers of food were required to file reports on which pesticides were applied during food production.

3. There were a data base available with information about all pesticides in use.

4. Cooperative agreements were made about pesticide use with foreign countries that export food to the United States.

There is no way for us ordinary shoppers to know whether unlabeled fruit is domestic or imported, and if it is imported there is no way to tell whether it comes from Chile, Mexico, or New Zealand. Merchants who sell fruit know and should post signs. Ask for this information at your supermarket.

MEAT INSPECTION FOR PESTICIDES

Meat and fish contaminated with high levels of pesticides may get to our plates without a check anywhere along the line. Animal-derived foods are the major source of pesticide residues stored in human fat. I wrote about that in the first edition of this book. The same holds true more than twenty years later.

It is the job of the Food Safety and Inspection Services (FSIS) of the United States Department of Agriculture to see that meat and poultry products are free of illegal residues. The Department of Agriculture's own Office of the Inspector General reported in 1988 that an audit of the FSIS revealed that it does not even routinely test for about 80 percent of the pesticides that could be present.[44] The inspector general's report also said:

- Investigations of illegal pesticide residues were ineffective in twenty-two of twenty-eight cases reviewed. The FSIS couldn't locate the producer (in twelve cases), failed to take follow-up samples (in nine cases), and "allowed the adulterated product to enter commerce when it would have been possible to prevent it" (in three cases).

- When residues of chemicals the FSIS wasn't looking for turned up, it frequently failed to evaluate them. It also lost records of pesticide violations and didn't collect residue tests within the time needed to make the tests valid and to stop distribution of the product.
- Routine testing was dropped for eleven meat producers who agreed to take extra precautions against illegal residues. Eight of the eleven never fully complied.

Are pesticide residue tolerances safe?

The Environmental Protection Agency in 1985 asked the National Research Council to study the pesticide residue risk situation. The NRC is the principal operating agency of the National Academy of Sciences and the National Academy of Engineering. The seventeen-member committee appointed included experts on toxicology, regulatory law, medicine, economics, plant protection, and agriculture.[45]

The committee considered the Delaney Amendment (which states that no cancer-causing agents shall be added to foods) of the Federal Food, Drug, and Cosmetic Act as it applied to pesticide residues. It concluded that strict adherence to the Delaney Amendment would require rescinding 51 percent of current tolerances for pesticides.

The committee found 31 cases in which the EPA allows a pesticide to be used on crops destined for processing even though these pesticides are believed to concentrate in processed foods and have been found to cause cancer in laboratory animals.

The committee identified 778 additional cases in which the residues of one or more pesticides posing potential cancer risks are likely to be present in certain processed foods. In many of these foods—particularly those that involve removing water or oils during processing—pesticide residues will concentrate, making them subject to the Delaney Amendment prohibition. However, the committee noted that the EPA lacks the required data on the carcinogenicity of many pesticides, as well as on which pesticides concentrate in processed foods and which do not.

The NRC committee concluded that the zero-tolerance residue for cancer-causing agents mandated by the Delaney Amendment is almost impossible to implement. A chemical's ability to cause cancer is particularly difficult to assess, the committee commented. The Delaney Amendment does not specify how a chemical's ability to "induce cancer" should be defined. For regulatory purposes, the EPA currently interprets the law to prohibit in processed foods concentrated levels of pesticides that cause cancer in animals or humans. The great majority of chemicals characterized by the EPA as cancer-causing have been identified through animal rather than human studies.

The committee found that about 90 percent of the total potential cancer-causing risk from the 28 compounds it studied intensively could be traced to pesticides registered before 1978. While the EPA has strictly applied the Delaney Amendment to pesticides registered after 1978, the agency has yet to apply it to those approved earlier.

The committee concluded that a uniform *negligible-risk standard,* defined as an estimated cancer risk of one additional case of cancer for every million people exposed, would achieve greater risk reduction and yet would impose fewer restrictions on agriculture than would the strict enforcement of the Delaney Amendment.

Considered in isolation from benefits provided by these compounds, the application of a single negligible-risk standard would require revoking 32 percent of the currently approved crop uses, or tolerances, for the 28 pesticides studied by the committee. Strict adherence to the Delaney Amendment would require rescinding 51 percent of current tolerances.

"Our report does not address *actual* exposure to potentially carcinogenic pesticide residues or the safety of individual foods," said Ray Thornton, president of the University of Arkansas and chairman of the Research Council committee. "We were only asked to look at levels of pesticide residues *allowed* under current federal laws and regulations. The key word here is *allowed.* Our analysis applies conservative EPA methods for calculating exposure to residues, including the assumption that pesticides are present in foods at their legal maximum. We do not believe this is true for the great majority of foods, but data on actual residue levels present on foods as eaten are limited."

The committee also cautioned that potential dietary cancer risks—though small—are only one of several possible environmental and health risks posed by pesticides.

Because the EPA has yet to revoke the registrations for the older, more carcinogenic pesticides, environmentalists have denounced the agency's decision to follow the negligible-risk standard.[46]

THE OTHER VIEW OF RESIDUES

Chemist Joseph Rosen of Rutgers's food science department points out that tolerance levels were initially established not because scientists had concluded these amounts were too low to cause cancer or mutations, but on the basis of toxicity. That is, the chemicals—intended in most cases to kill insects or microorganisms—were tested to find out how much of them laboratory animals could eat and still survive.

Maximum tolerance levels that included substantial safety margins were then set for humans. The cancer risk explored in the NRC study was based on what could be expected if people actually consumed these maximum amounts.

Rosen says that Rutgers chemists studied fruits and vegetables to find just how much residue was on them.

"The chemicals we tested for include most of the known or suspected carcinogens and mutagens that are used on these crops, plus a few other pesticides. . . . The largest amount of residue they found on the most samples," Rosen reports, "was the fungicide benomyl, which the chemists detected on eighteen of the twenty-five samples of peaches, but at levels ranging from 0.25 to 3.48 ppm, with an average of 0.8 ppm or about 5 percent of the tolerance level of 15 ppm. The researchers also found benomyl on five of the twenty-five apple samples, ranging from a trace to 0.59 ppm. The tolerance level for apples is 7 ppm. A trace was also detected on one sample of tomatoes, for which the tolerance is 5 ppm."[47]

Benomyl, by the way, is a carbamate (see page 12) and is highly toxic when ingested.[48]

Alar, the apple-growth regulator and a particular focus of alarm in 1988–89, could be detected in only one of twenty-five apple samples, at 0.32 ppm; the established tolerance level is 20 ppm.

Rosen says these residues "are something the intelligent person should not be worried about."

Bruce Ames, Ph.D., who developed the Ames Test to detect mutagens and thus potential cancer-causing agents, is another scientist who has become vocal against "alarmists" about pesticides and cancer-causing chemicals in food. Dr. Ames and Lois Swirsky Gold, his colleague at the department of biochemistry, University of California at Berkeley, maintain:

"Regulation of low dose exposure to chemicals based on animal cancer tests may not result in significant reduction of human cancer, because we are exposed to millions of different chemicals—almost all natural—and it is not feasible to test all of them."[49]

Does Professor Rosen, Ames, Gold, or anyone from the National Research committee know how much of a cancer-causing agent causes cancer?

Do they know what happens if we should eat vegetables and fruits with minute amounts of different pesticide residues in the same meal?

Grapes alone, according to Cesar Chavez, are sprayed with five different pesticides.[50]

We certainly hope they can answer those questions soon. In the meantime, what can we do?

WHAT CAN WE DO?

We cannot depend upon government regulations and inspectors to protect us. Even if we had ten times the number of safeguards and inspectors, chances are that some pesticide-contaminated food would still get through.

What is the answer? Better education, of course; but this is not easy to achieve.

If farmers were to handle pesticides as the government and its extension services recommend, they would all need college degrees in chemistry and the consciences of saints. The mixing and handling directions for many pesticides are complicated, especially for farm help, many of whom are illiterate. Such safety precautions as going to a dump and burying the containers are time-consuming, to say the least. Keeping from the market food that is known to be pesticide-contaminated means a great financial loss, and is much to ask of a person who must scratch a living from the land.

Some farmers are doing their own testing for pesticide residues to reassure customers that their crops are safe. Maine farmers, for example, have a program to test for twenty-four pesticides commonly used on their $115 million potato crop.

If they can't convince you of safety, however, they can always use the money angle. Chemicals are a substitute for labor; removing more farm chemicals for the market would force farmers to add more workers in the field and would cause higher production costs.[51]

What can we do?

- We can urge the Congress to appropriate additional funds for increased testing and monitoring of pesticides.
- We can urge federal testing for any pesticides that may not be covered by all screening programs now in effect.
- We can urge the government to inspect foods more diligently for unsafe residues and ensure that imported products meet domestic safety standards.
- We can ask the president to establish a single federal agency assigned to ensure food safety and provide uniformity and consistency in the development and enforcement of safety laws governing the ways in which foods are grown, processed, and distributed. And until such an agency is formed, we can urge that the EPA, the FDA, and the USDA expedite health-risk studies for all pesticides now in use, with separate and equal attention to effects on children and adults.

NEW SUBSTITUTES FOR CHEMICAL PESTICIDES

We must also encourage new methods of pest control. There is great incentive today to do so because European countries—which will become one market in 1992—are working toward a 50 percent reduction in the use of pesticides, and it has Americans worried. Disharmony in pesticide regulations between the United States and various European countries could harm our agricultural exports.[52]

Furthermore, the repeated use of so many pesticides and herbicides on the same land has made a lot of these chemicals ineffective.[53]

The fact is that with all our deadly pesticides, we have not destroyed our insect pests. We have just as many bugs today as when we began applying DDT, and the ones we have are rapidly gaining resistance to the chemicals. And we have succeeded in killing off the natural enemies of these pests. It may be hard to raise sympathy for bats, for instance, but the animals are generally useful and harmless. Insect-eating bats are among the most susceptible of all animals to the poisons.

BETTER TIMING

David Call, dean of Cornell University's College of Agricultural and Life Sciences, said that apple growers in New York State spray fungicides, insecticides, and miticides as well as daminozide on their trees eight to fourteen times a season, in part because the trees and fruit are threatened by insects and disease. Dr. Call maintained, however, that much of this heavy use of chemicals is for cosmetic purposes or because of federal or state standards limiting the amount of harmless insect parts that may appear on fruit.[54]

He said the amount of pesticides used on apples and other crops could be reduced substantially by the use of integrated pest management, which calls for a more judicious use of chemicals in smaller quantities, along with natural enemies of crop pests.

NEW METHOD OF GETTING RID OF PESTICIDES IN WATER

Agricultural pesticide spray operations generate large volumes of low-concentration mixed-composition wastes in water. Improper disposal of these residues may lead to groundwater contamination. A recently developed technology that adds ozone to waste water greatly reduced the concentration of three pesticides. Atrazine, cyanazine, and metolachlor, at concentrations of 17, 30, and 82 ppm respectively, were decreased to less than 5 ppm. This process was not as effective for paraquat, in which concentrations were decreased from 40 to 18 ppm. Adding the ozone to the waste water eliminated herbicidal activity and provided products that were more readily degraded in the soil than was the parent material.[55]

At the time of this writing, the USDA is about to ask Congress for more than $40 million to fund research and to institute programs to prevent pesticides and nitrates from entering groundwater.

Richard Amerman, assistant to the director of the USDA's Agriculture Research Services, said: "The first part of the program will be fundamental research to develop new technology. The second will be to educate farmers and implement technology already developed to keep pesticides out of the groundwater. The third will be to establish a data base that contains water conditions and pesticide use and characteristics—how rapidly a pesticide breaks down . . . how much is used by farmers and so forth."[56]

Why hasn't a data base been established before?

"We did have a data base in the 1970s but the funds were cut back by Congress and the program was shut down," Amerman explained.

He said that because funds are limited, the program is going to concentrate on the midwestern corn and soybean belt, where the most significant problems seem to occur.

NATURAL PESTICIDES

Seeds, leaves, roots, and other plant parts can produce their own pesticides and weed killers. Natural plant compounds that interfere with insect growth, development, reproduction, and communication are producing exciting new chemical compounds that may yield selective, environmentally harmless products for insect control.[57] Pyrethrins, for example, are derived from chrysanthemums and have been used for many years in "nontoxic to humans and animals" household pesticides.

A word of caution: just because a substance is a natural pesticide in a plant or an insect does not mean it is harmless. Researchers must proceed with caution.[58]

Naturally occurring toxicants (natural pesticides) in plants have caused problems in animals and humans throughout history. Early Americans had severe difficulties in their westward movement due to the dreaded illness "milk sickness," which was known as early as the Revolutionary War. Milk sickness was contracted by drinking milk from cows that had fed on the toxic plant white snakeroot.

Plants that contain naturally occurring toxicants also may make up some of our common food. It is widely accepted that plants produce such chemicals to defend themselves from insects, microbes, and other plant pests. Many of these chemicals are produced by plants in a general response to many types of external stimuli. If plants are bred to increase the levels of these natural pesticides, an inadvertent result may be increased toxicity for humans and animals.[59]

For example, a new variety of insect-resistant potato had to be withdrawn from the market because of acute toxicity to humans caused by high levels of the teratogens solanine and chaconine, which are not normally present in potatoes. Similarly, a new variety of insect-resistant celery recently introduced widely in the United States caused outbreaks of skin rash in produce workers owing to a concentration of the carcinogen 8-methoxypsoralen of 9,000 parts per billion (ppb) rather than the usual 900 ppb.

USING INSECT DEFENSES

Just as plants have natural defenses against pests, so do insects. These natural insect products are being studied for use as crop pesticides. Many species of insects secrete malodorous *allomones,* which can disrupt the attack behavior of an enemy.[60]

And natural insect attractant may also be used to confound the bugs. For example, up to one hundred tons of chemical pesticides now applied to New York vineyards to control grape berry moth could be replaced by small plastic ties impregnated with tiny amounts of natural sex attractant (pheromones), Cornell biologists have found. The insect pheromones confuse male moths and disrupt mating.[61]

Sexual lures are also being used to save pickles. A box trap and a newly synthesized pheromone may help farmers in North and South Carolina cut down to almost half the amount of manufactured chemical pesticides currently being used to combat pickle worms.

The appearance of male moths in traps would signal cucumber growers when pesticides are truly needed.

Growers, at present, begin spraying as soon as nighttime temperatures reach sixty°F. Preliminary tests show that growers could get the same protection using the pheromone traps and about half as much spraying as they could using the conventional seasonal temperature-based spraying approach.

NATURAL PREDATORS

William M. Metterhouse, director, Division of Plant Industry, New Jersey Department of Agriculture, Trenton, says the natural enemies of parasites, flies, and beetles can be used as "pesticides." There are insect diseases such as viruses, fungi, and bacteria that are harmless to humans and animals but lethal to certain crop pests. Little insectaries are being established in New Jersey. When beetles lay their eggs on the snap bean crop, the beneficial parasites grown in the insectaries are released and they kill the beetle eggs. This method has been able to control 80 to 90 percent of the beetle populations.[62]

Not only does introducing the natural enemies of pests reduce the need to spray agricultural chemicals, but the reduced spraying then allows the beneficial native insects to reestablish themselves.

MICROENCAPSULATION AND CONTROLLED RELEASE

The technique of microencapsulation—surrounding toxic pesticides in tiny "bubbles"—looked promising in the early 1970s, according to researchers at the 1989 American Chemical Society meeting in Miami, but the "coated killers" never really became popular because they cost more than conventional pesticides.

Microencapsulation techniques also can provide time-released pesticides, hormones, and sexual pheromones. The capsules disintegrate at different rates over a period of time. Microencapsulated pesticides are safer for farmers to handle and don't travel in air, water, and soil as much as do conventional applications. As the government regulations get stricter, microencapsulation and controlled release may become more desirable, despite their higher costs.[63]

GENETICALLY ALTERED PESTICIDE

Biotechnology—the science of manipulating DNA, the basic blueprint of cells—also has tremendous possibilities (some say both good and bad). Researchers at University Green, Middleton, Wisconsin, for example, are using genes from two different organisms to create plants that are resistant to insect pests.[64]

In July 1989, the federal government allowed researchers at Cornell University in Ithaca to conduct open-air test spraying of a genetically engineered virus used as an insecticide.[65] Researchers say the test is important because it could remove one of the toughest hurdles they face in their quest to develop a viral pesticide that works as quickly as chemicals.

The Foundation for Economic Trends, a Washington, D.C., environmental group, has opposed the release of all such organisms since 1983, when it filed suit to stop a California company from testing an altered bacterium. The foundation feels there is no way to assess whether an experiment would be dangerous.

Natural viruses have been used since 1946, but they are slow to act compared with chemical pesticides. They also may stay in the environment attacking benevolent insects after they have wiped out the pests. The Cornell researchers hope to solve the latter problem by removing a single gene that causes the viruses to grow a protective coating, without which they die quickly in the open. The ultimate goal is a fast-acting virus that dies soon after leaving the pest's body.

One fear is that the virus would recombine with naturally occurring viruses, gaining a protective coat from its natural cousins but retaining its lethal ability to cause chaos in an insect's system.

SHEEP ARE REPLACING DEFOLIANTS

Sheep and teams of woodsmen have replaced chemical defoliants along Oregon's Pacific coast as government foresters use safer methods for cleaning brush from slopes for new forests. Before, the type of defoliants used included 2,4,5-T, 2,4-D, and picloram. Agent Orange, the defoliant used in the Vietnam War, was a mixture of 2,4,5-T and 2,4-D.

In 1979, because of protests and the discovery that women in this region suffered an unusually high rate of miscarriages, the Environmental Protection Agency banned the use of 2,4,5-T.[66]

THE VACUUM-CLEANER APPROACH

A vacuum cleaner was mounted aboard a grape-harvesting machine to test the practicality of sucking insects off the vines. The machine is working well not only on grapes but on strawberries and lettuce. It has cut the use of pesticides on Salinas Valley strawberry and lettuce fields.[67]

ORGANIC FARMING

Some of the largest California lettuce, fruit, and wine growers started to go "organic" in the late 1980s. The *New York Times* described the farming techniques of a Vienna, Virginia, woman and her children who used "natural pesticides and fertilizers" within hearing distance of Dulles International Airport.[68]

Mrs. Tony Newcomb and her daughters and their husbands planted a twenty-eight-acre farm. They used only natural fertilizers, disease-resistant plant varieties, and limited use of natural bacteria and pesticides derived from plants. In addition predator insects like ladybugs, lacewings, praying mantises, and chalic wasps were allowed to flourish and devour unwanted bugs. The Newcombs also did a lot of overplanting and successive plantings to compensate for pest damage. They used the natural fertilizer from horse farms in the area; the neighbors didn't object to the stench because they got pesticide-free eggs and vegetables.

As more farmers sell "organics," how can you be sure you are really buying pesticide- and herbicide-free produce or meat? Some states have definitions of "organic" but the definitions vary. Texas certifies organic farm produce and the products carry a TDA Certified Organic label.

Conventional industry and government propaganda holds that the United States has the "safest food supply in the world." And most supermarkets, with their aisles of colorful processed food, overflowing freezers, and meticulously arranged fresh produce, reinforce this notion for millions of consumers every day.

HOW DO YOU KNOW YOUR FOOD IS SAFE FROM HARMFUL PESTICIDE?

A lot of what's sold isn't safe at all. Pesticide-contaminated food is a topic of growing concern as overuse, misuse, and abuse of these toxic chemicals escalates. According to a recent survey conducted by the Food Marketing Institute, "Three out of four consumers consider residues such as pesticides and herbicides to be a serious health hazard." Unfortunately, the very fact that health-conscious consumers are trying to eat more fresh fruits and vegetables compounds the problem because those are the produce most likely to be contaminated.

New York in 1983 issued regulations that would have required restaurants, hotels, shopping malls, schools, public parks, libraries, hospitals, trains, bus stations, airports, office buildings, and department stores, among other establishments, to post signs saying they were using pesticides. A state judge, however, overturned these regulations because he said that the department overstepped the authority granted to it by the Legislature.[69]

Californians came up with similar regulations that became law in 1989. According to the Safe Drinking Water and Toxic Enforcement Act, better known as Proposition 65, a business must warn the public if it knowingly exposes them to any substance that poses a significant risk of cancer or birth defects.

The state of California was charged with coming up with a list of known carcinogens and reproductive toxins and then took upon itself the task of defining "significant risk": 1 excess cancer case (1 more than usual) per 100,000 people reasonably exposed throughout their lifetimes. Under the law no warning is required unless a chemical is present in an amount that exceeds the *significant risk* threshold. The State has now listed some 250 chemicals and has set standards or allowable doses for another 50 widely used ones.

Substances on the state of California's list include alcoholic beverages, tobacco smoke, plastic, gasoline, benzene arsenic, lead, asbestos, vinyl chloride, chromium, urethane in red wine, nitroso compounds in bacon and other cured meats, and formaldehyde in everything from toothpastes to mobile homes.[70]

Bruce Ames, who is a member of the California governor's advisory panel, has become one of the law's most outspoken critics. He said, "Proposition 65 is based on the assumption that these chemicals are dangerous, but all science points against pollutants having much to do with public health." (Read chapter 7 and see if you agree with him.) Ames called "wildly exaggerated the commonly accepted view that 3 to 4 percent of all cancers in the United States are due to environmental exposures. Occupational exposures may account for some," he says, "pollution probably for none."

Ames maintains that in the cases where half the chemicals tested, natural as well as synthetic, turn out to be labeled "carcinogens," either the tests are in error or the carcinogens used at the dosages identified are just not that dangerous.

Ames is often quoted as urging the public to ignore pollution, which he considers a red herring, and focus on what he considers the real culprits, such as too much fat in the diet, overexposure to sunlight, and the use of tobacco.

THE SUPERMARKET PERSPECTIVE

What are supermarkets doing? Kings in Short Hills, New Jersey, is one of a chain of eighteen high-quality supermarkets. They not only have a great variety of fruits and vegetables, but also offer cooking and educational classes in their own cooking school right in the store. They have a certified dietician with offices on the premises. Rob Bildner, president of RLB Food Distributors, is a member of the family that began Kings.[71]

At a store lecture in 1989, he gave the supermarket owner's view of the alarm over pesticides in food. "We see our role [is] to find alternatives. We have a very vigorous approach. We work with our growers and ask about the fertilizers, insecticides, and fungicides they use.

"Our goal is to see the elimination of all chemicals down the road. . . . But if that were done today, practically speaking, 90 percent of the produce wouldn't be here. It is practically impossible at this stage in our society and our economy. We hope to change reliance on chemically intensive produce to more organically based produce over the next ten years.

"We buy sixty percent of our strawberries from Driscoll of California, depending on the season. Driscoll is one of the finer strawberries, bigger and sweeter and more expensive than other strawberries. The Driscoll Company has gone into a program now to eliminate use of pesticides."

Bildner said that many customers feel that they don't care what the government says, they don't want *any* detectable residues on their fruit.

He said he personally believes that "no detectable levels" of pesticides means that the crops are safe. But, he said, because of the concern of the customers, the chain's position has been not only to meet government standards, but to go beyond them.

Bildner said that Superior, a large California grower of grapes, nectarines, and plums, has a major laboratory in which it does its own testing for pesticide residues, so the fruit is tested before leaving California. The fruit has a seal on the box stating that it meets both the state of California's and federal standards: "The Superior people are smart because they recognize the consumers' concern about chemicals. It's a million dollars' worth of public relations."

Bildner said organically grown fruits and vegetables are sold at Kings but the market can't get a sufficient supply.

"There just isn't enough to go around. Organics must be certified by the state in which they are grown or by an organization of organic farmers. California began by saying produce could be labeled 'organic' if the ground in which it was grown was free of pesticides and fertilizers for one year. California is now requiring the ground be free of pesticides and herbicides for three years, a requirement Texas has to certify produce as 'organic.'

"Products that are grown free of pesticides but [in land that] hasn't been free of the chemicals for the required time are called *traditional crops*," Bildner continued.

Some supermarket chains are testing for pesticides as a competitive weapon, Bildner said, a situation he felt could undermine consumer confidence and raise prices.

"If we ever do testing, we would want to do it in a responsible way. It would not be possible to test for 300 substances, just five or ten. Screening for all of them would be too costly because it is very expensive to test—about $300 a test.

"We have 40,000 cases of produce delivered a week in 18 stores. Who would pay for the testing program? You would. Some growers will do it but the supermarket margins are so small, the consumers would have to pay for it. It would cost us 10 times our food prices to do one case of produce."

He said that 35 percent of Kings' produce is foreign; that most growers in Mexico are American companies; and that Chile is a sophisticated user of pesticides. He claimed that if fruits and vegetables were held up for more testing at the borders, shelf life would be lost.

WHAT CAN YOU DO TO SAFEGUARD YOUR FOOD AGAINST PESTICIDE CONTAMINATION?

- Wash all produce, even that which comes prepackaged. Water will remove some pesticide traces. Scrub with a soft brush. Do not use detergents, which may be harmful to the mucous lining of the stomach and intestines and have perfumes and artificial colors. If you feel you must use more than water, use a soap, which is easier to rinse off than is a detergent. Rinse thoroughly.
- Peel fruits and vegetables when feasible.
- Pull off the outer leaves of lettuce and cabbage, where pesticides concentrate. For the same reason, trim the leaves and tops of celery.
- Buy American. Some imported foods may have twice the amount of pesticides that home-grown have.
- Buy in season to avoid the pesticides that make strawberries in January possible.

- Beware of perfection. The best-looking fruit or vegetable is not always the best-tasting, and it may have been treated with a cosmetic wax that holds moisture and pesticide residues.
- Buy organic produce for fruits and vegetables that your children eat.
- Trim all fat off meat and poultry. It is better for you anyway, and many of the chemicals concentrate in fat.
- Don't eat liver. Besides being too high in cholesterol, a lot of the chemicals concentrate in the liver.
- Stores are supposed to post signs to inform you when produce has been waxed. I've never seen one.
- Don't bite into orange or lemon peels unless you scrub them thoroughly.
- Grow your own.

HOW YOU CAN PROTECT YOUSELF FROM IMPROPER USE OF PESTICIDES IN YOUR HOME

I shudder to think of the many times I sprayed my own backyard to kill ants and used insecticide on the rose bushes while my husband watered the lawn and the children and dog played nearby. So that you won't make the same mistakes, or any others with pesticides, here is some advice:

- Read the label and follow the directions. Reread them each time before using the pesticide. Take the advice seriously. If it says to wear rubber gloves, for instance, do so!
- Use the right pesticide at the right time. Try to pick the least poisonous for the job. Measure accurately.
- Work in a well-ventilated area.
- Keep pesticides out of reach of children. In one instance, a year-old infant found lindane tablets for a vaporizer under the sink in her home. She ate four or five of them and died at the hospital shortly afterward. In the same city, an eighteen-month-old boy swallowed half a lindane tablet found on the floor of his family car. He died twelve hours later.
- Do not spray pesticides of any kind anywhere if you are pregnant or around a pregnant woman.

- When spraying inside the home to control flying insects, cover all food and utensils. After spraying, leave the room immediately and close the door. Do not reenter for half an hour or longer. Aquariums as well as birds, dogs, cats, and other pets must be removed before you spray.
- Outside, remove or cover food and water containers used by pets.
- Do not contaminate fish ponds or streams.
- Always keep pesticides in their original containers. Make sure they are tightly closed and plainly labeled. Never put a pesticide in an empty food or drink container of any kind.
- Never smoke, drink, or chew gum while handling pesticides.
- Avoid inhaling sprays, dusts, or vapors.
- Have soap, water, and a towel available. Should you spill concentrated pesticide on yourself, wash immediately.
- When you have finished using a pesticide, wash hands and face thoroughly and remove contaminated clothing before smoking or eating.
- Work clothes should be laundered before they are used again.
- Be careful about your shoes. Sometimes they soak up the pesticide; if they do, throw them out.
- Store pesticides and pesticide equipment in a locked cabinet or room that is cool, dry, and well ventilated.
- Never store pesticides with or near food, medicine, or cleaning supplies.
- Some pesticides may have vapors that can be absorbed by nearby containers.
- Be careful in disposing of containers. Do not burn them. Wrap them in several layers of newspaper and place them in a trash can just before the trash is collected. Until then, lock them up.
- Purchase only what you need for one season.
- If you have a special sensitivity to pesticides, consult a physician and, if necessary, avoid further exposure to the offending chemicals.
- If you experience headache, nausea, or blurred vision, or if you accidentally swallow any pesticide, call a physician immediately. Read the label to him. If necessary, go to a doctor's office or hospital and take the empty container with you.

3 ✎ Your Food—Plus What? Deliberate and Accidental Hidden Ingredients

A lovely nineteen-year-old college sophomore with everything to live for was having a wonderful time at a college dormitory party. She had a history of childhood allergies and had had systemic reactions after eating eggs, poppy seeds, peanuts, peas, or fish; other than that, she was in perfect health. As she chatted with classmates, she picked up and took two bites of a cookie that had as a hidden ingredient peanut oil. She realized that she was beginning to have an allergy attack and took a pill she kept with her for just such an occasion.

The pill didn't work—at least not fast enough. She collapsed and her friends rushed her to the campus health service. When she arrived, she had no pulse or respiration. A physician administered two doses of epinephrine, a stimulant, and attempted heart-lung resuscitation, but to no avail. The young woman was dead.[1]

At another college, a co-ed, a year younger, also had a history of allergy to nuts. She was eating at a nearby campus restaurant with friends when she took two bites of chili containing the hidden ingredient, peanut butter. She became short of breath. She refused to go to a hospital and instead asked to be taken to the home of a friend whose father was a physician. The doctor administered epinephrine and called the rescue squad, but the girl died in the ambulance on the way to the hospital.[2]

Allergic reactions to hidden ingredients in processed foods or in restaurant meals are common.

A doctor's daughter sat down to breakfast one morning, poured a bowl of crisp corn flakes, added some milk, then swallowed several spoonfuls. She drank no other beverage and ate no other food. Within minutes, her uvula, the piece of flesh that hangs down in the back of the throat, had swelled. It took great effort for her to move her limbs and she felt extremely fatigued. An allergist tested her skin for sensitivity to corn and to cow's milk, but she showed no allergic reaction to either.

The source of her sudden spell of illness remained a mystery until she sat down to supper one day and took a bite of instant mashed potatoes. She suffered the same attack of throat swelling, extreme weakness, and fatigue. Again the allergist tested the patient's skin, this time for potato extract, and again the results were negative.

Puzzled by the young woman's symptoms, the allergist examined the labels on the box of corn flakes and the box of potatoes. The corn flakes she had ingested had been treated with BHA (butylated hydroxyanisole) to preserve freshness. The package of potatoes the young woman had eaten from listed BHT (butylated hydroxytoluene, a relative of BHA) as a preservative and antimold agent. All the girl's symptoms disappeared when she stopped eating foods that contained BHA and BHT.[3]

Another case difficult to diagnose involved a middle-aged man who came to the Headache Clinic at Montefiore Hospital in the Bronx, New York. He suffered from severe headaches on Thanksgiving, Christmas, and New Year's Day. The possibility of a psychological cause, of course, was strong because on these occasions he always ate and drank a lot and his mother-in-law came for dinner. The main dish was inevitably turkey.

It took several years to pinpoint the turkey as the indirect cause of the headaches. It turned out that the patient was allergic to penicillin; and, although he lived in New York, he always ate New Jersey turkeys that had been fed on a mash containing penicillin.[4]

From the fertilizer put on the ground to the "flavorings" and "colorings" in processed foods, there are additives in your meal.

The FDA knows of more than 3,000 additives found in our foods but has a data base with information on only 1,586 of them.[5] The majority of food additives are believed to be safe so long as dosages do not exceed those set by the Food and Drug Administration, although many scientists—including former FDA commissioner James L. Goddard—say we really don't know enough about their safety.[6]

Chemicals are added to food for a variety of reasons:

- *As Coloring Agents.* The natural coloring materials in foods may be intensified, modified, or stabilized by the addition of natural coloring materials, certified food dyes, or derived colors. These chemicals that enhance the appearance of food are considered important for the aesthetic value they add and the psychological effect they have on our food consumption habits.
- *As Antispoilants.* Chemicals may be used to help prevent microbiological spoilage and chemical deterioration. There is a growing preference for these food additives.
- *As Flavoring Agents.* In number—2,112—flavoring additives probably exceed all other intentional chemical food additives combined. Of these, 502 are natural and 1,610 synthetic.
- *As Agents to Improve Functional Properties.* Chemicals in this classification act as thickening, firming, and maturing agents or affect the colloidal properties of foods by jelling, emulsifying, foaming, or suspending. Calcium salts, for example, help the texture of canned tomatoes by preventing them from becoming too soft.
- *As Processing Aids.* Sanitizing agents, metal binding compounds, antifoaming agents, chemicals that prevent fermentation, and chemicals that remove extraneous materials are grouped in this classification. Examples are silicones to prevent foam formation in wine fermentation, and citric acid to prevent oxidation rancidity.
- *As Moisture Content Controls.* Chemicals sometimes are used to increase or decrease the moisture content in food products. For instance, glycerin is approved for use in marshmallows as a humectant to retain soft texture. Calcium silicate is frequently added to table salt to prevent caking due to moisture in the air.

- *As Acid-alkaline Controls*. Various acids, alkalis, and salts may be added to food to establish a desired pH, or acid-alkaline balance. Phosphoric acid in soft drinks and citrate salts in fruit jellies are examples of this chemical control of acid-alkaline balance.
- *As Physiologic Activity Controls*. The chemicals in this group are usually added to fresh foods to serve as ripeners or anti-metabolic agents. Examples of applications for this purpose are ethylene, used to hasten the ripening of bananas, and maleic hydrazide, used to prevent potatoes from sprouting.
- *As Nutrition Supplements*. The use of vitamins, minerals, and amino acids has become widespread. The enrichment of cereal foods alone provides 12 to 23 percent of the daily supply of thiamine, niacin, and iron, and 10 percent of riboflavin recommended for human consumption.

Most of the time, the consumer is unaware that these additives are in products in the supermarket. Take some random examples:

Uncle Ben's Country Inn Herbed Rice Au Gratin® has a front label that says: "Inspired by the 'Finest Inn' " and "now more cheese." Uncle Ben's ingredient list reads: "contains enriched par-boiled long grain rice (BHT added as a preservative), dried mozzarella, swiss, parmesan cheeses (milk culture, enzymes, salt), wild rice, dehydrated vegetables (carrots, parsley, spinach, leeks), partially hydrogenated vegetable oil (soybean and/or cottonseed), sugar, natural flavor, monosodium glutamate, salt, nonfat dry milk, modified food starch, butter, chicken fat, dry chicken meat, silicon dioxide, mono and disodium phosphate, xanthan gum, whey, guar gum, maltodextrin, buttermilk, hydrolyzed cereal solids, extract corn, malted barley, chicken broth, turmeric, artificial flavor, sage, tricalcium phosphate, mono and diglycerides, citric acid, BHA, propyl gallate, sodium sulfite and sodium bisulfite as preservatives." (Nowhere does the label tell you how much sodium is in the product, but rest assured an ocean would be envious of the salt content.)

Reddi wip® (made by Beatrice Cheese, Inc.), which says on the label "instant real whipped cream," has as ingredients an ultra-pasteurized blend of cream, nonfat milk solids, sugar, corn syrup, mono- and diglycerides, artificial flavor, carrageenan, whipping gas (nitrous oxide).

Sara Lee's® frozen cream cheesecake contains cream cheese (pasteurized milk and cream, cheese cultures, salt, carob bean gum, guar gum), sugar, fresh whole eggs, corn syrup, enriched flour (with niacin, iron, thiamine mononitrate (Vitamin B_1), riboflavin (vitamin B_2), light cream, partially hydrogenated vegetable shortening (soybean/or cottonseed oils), whole wheat flour, sour cream, vanilla, skim milk, salt, modified starch, molasses, xanthan gum, baking powder (baking soda, monocalcium phosphate), carob bean gum, cinnamon, carrageenan, guar gum. The label reads "no artificial flavors or preservatives."

Without additives, Herbed Rice Au Gratin® and Reddi wip® would be utterly impossible to manufacture. Without additives, Sara Lee's® cheesecake, because of limited shelf life, might be commercially unfeasible.

In addition to those ingredients listed on the labels, there are ingredients in products that do not have to be listed.

- *Standard Foods*. For more than three hundred foods—including ice cream, catsup, and mayonnaise—no ingredients need be listed. Processors follow the standard chemical recipes written out by the government. The manufacturer is given the option of choosing among many alternative standard chemicals, and only if he substitutes or adds a nonstandard chemical or uses Yellow No. 5 or No. 6 (both well-known allergens) must he indicate the fact on the label. Ice cream, for example, which can have some thirty additives, need not list ingredients on the label. In products such as canned fruit and gelatin desserts, the processor need only state *"artificial coloring"* or *"artifical flavoring"* without specifically identifying it, again with the exception of Yellow No. 5 and No. 6.
- *Processing Chemicals*. The law does not require that chemicals added in small amounts during processing, such as calcium bromate (a maturing agent for dough), be included on the label.

- *Residues from Agricultural Chemicals, Antibiotics, Hormones, and Other Unintentional Additives.* These are not listed on labels, but they can have an effect on those who ingest them with their meals. In chapter 4, on meat and poultry, you will read about hidden hormones and antibiotics in your food, which have been deposited there from animal feed and treatments. Chapter 2 contains a discussion of pesticide residues in food.
- *Migration from Packaging.* Allergy, cancer, and mutagenicity may result from packaging.[7] There are several hundred chemicals used in formulating food-packaging materials that might become additives; the basic glass, film paper, metal, cloth, or wood plus the sizing and coating material; the plasticizers, the adhesives, the dyes and printing inks; the solvents, germicides, antioxidants, and other miscellaneous chemicals associated with them. The Food Additives Amendment of 1958 gave the Food and Drug Administration the responsibility of making sure that indirect additives in foods, including those that migrate into them from packaging materials, be regulated to assure human safety. The FDA is supposed to be given the following information about each new packaging material:

1. Whether or not it gets into the food.
2. How much may get in.
3. Whether that amount is safe for people to ingest.

The FDA demanded proof that organo-tin compounds are safe for food packaging. They are not (see page 184), and they were not used. On the other hand, many packages are made of plastic. Plastics behave differently with various foodstuffs. A plastic container that is not attacked by sugar or acid may be fine for jams. But the unsuspecting housewife may decide to reuse the empty container to collect drippings, unaware that certain toxic constituents may be extracted by the fat.[8] In 1971, it was discovered that plastic bags containing blood for transfusions released a toxic substance into the blood. It was an unexpected finding, happened upon by chance by a Baltimore researcher tracking down a substance in the blood of patients. If someone were to look, perhaps he too would find similar problems with plastic lid containers and wrappings for meat.

Another packaging material, lead solder, is worrisome. According to industry data in 1987, lead solder is used in about 6 percent of cans filled in the United States, down from 90 percent ten years ago. There are no figures for imported cans.[9]

It was revealed in September 1989 that bleached paper cartons holding milk and other food products can leach low levels of dioxin, a powerful cancer-causing agent.[10] The FDA tentatively estimated that the lifetime cancer risks would be less than one in a million from drinking milk in such cartons. In the meantime, paper manufacturers are working to get the dioxin out of paper board.

Medical diagnosis is always an educated guess, but with so many intentional and unintentional additives in our food, it is difficult—at times impossible—to link an ailment with "something" you ate.

SOMETHING YOU ATE?

An adverse reaction or sensitivity to a food means *any abnormal* reaction to a food or food additive that is eaten. Here are the basic categories:

- *Food Intolerance.* An adverse reaction to food due to such factors as enzyme deficiencies, contaminants or toxins, drug use, heredity, psychological disorder, and underlying disease. If you get indigestion from eating beans, that's an intolerance. The adverse reaction is usually caused by factors in the diet other than protein. One of the more common food intolerance reactions may be the result of the body's inability to digest lactose (milk sugar). Many people, particularly as they grow older, are deficient in the enzyme needed to process lactose.
- *Pharmacologic Food Reactions.* An adverse reaction to a chemical, found in a food or food additive, that produces a druglike effect; for instance: caffeine in coffee, causing the "jitters"; the amines in cheese, causing a headache.

The "Chinese restaurant syndrome," manifested by anxiety, flushed face, and pressure in the chest, has been shown to be caused by eating large amounts of the flavor enhancer MSG. Sulfite preservatives are known to have the potential to cause a serious attack of asthma and even death. An array of psychological and psychiatric diseases has been related to the diet. In addition, epileptic changes detected by EEGs have been reported to be associated with food sensitivity.[11]

- *Food Poisoning*. An adverse reaction caused by a food or food additive without your immune system being involved. Toxins (poisons or bacteria) may be either contained within the food or released by microorganisms or parasites contaminating the food.
- *Food Allergy*. Involves the immune system. If you are allergic to a food or food additive, your body's immune system over-reacts to it. The food or food additive may be harmless to others, but you suffer irritating, uncomfortable symptoms because you are hypersensitive to it. The word "allergy" is derived from two Greek words that can be roughly translated as "altered response."

The National Institute of Allergy and Infectious Diseases estimates that there are thirty-five million people in this country who have allergic reactions to substances that, in similar amounts, are apparently completely harmless to most people. The number of ailments diagnosed as allergies is undoubtedly going to rise as more is discovered about this group of diseases and as our environment becomes more complex.

It is difficult to recognize a food allergy because:

- Allergic reactions may be delayed from several hours to days after ingestion of the offending food.
- You may eat the food only once in awhile.
- You may be allergic to that food only at certain times.
- There may be an interaction between a food and a drug you are taking.
- The quantity of food eaten may influence the reaction.
- The cooking method may influence the reaction.
- There may be hidden additives and contaminants in the food, as pointed out above.

Symptoms of delayed sensitivity may include anything from muscle aches to mental symptoms, drowsiness, and confusion, all of which are also symptoms of many other, nonallergic ailments.

There is no doubt, however, about a food allergy when an anaphylactic attack occurs, such as the ones mentioned at the beginning of this chapter. It is an immediate, dramatic, life-threatening, generalized allergic reaction. It may involve any system of the body but usually affects the skin, nose, throat, lungs, stomach, heart, and blood vessels. The first signs may be a red, itchy rash and a feeling of warmth. These may be followed by light-headedness, shortness of breath or sneezing, a feeling of anxiety, stomach or uterine cramps, and/or vomiting and diarrhea. Foods frequently listed as the causes of anaphylaxis include peanuts, nuts, shellfish, eggs, and seeds.

Food allergens are usually proteins. The fact that neurotransmitters—the chemicals that send messages between nerve cells—in the brain are made from proteins suggests that brain allergies may exist.

Most of the allergens can still cause reactions even after they have undergone digestion. Recent studies in the United States indicate that proteins in cow's milk, eggs, peanuts, wheat, and soy are the most common food allergens. Others include shellfish, pork, corn, strawberries, tuna, chicken, chocolate, nuts, tomatoes, peas, oranges, and cabbage. But almost any food can be an allergen. Also, some people can become sensitive to the artificial coloring agents, vegetable gums, and other substances widely used in prepared foods. Cooking can reduce the effect of some protein allergens but may increase the effect of others.[12]

Sometimes an allergen is a food that has been eaten for many years without any ill effect. Unknown to the victim, the allergy has been developing slowly.

If symptoms of a food allergy appear quickly—during a meal or just after a specific food has been eaten—it is usually fairly easy to discover the responsible allergen. But if the reaction is delayed, then it is necessary to investigate, either by the process of elimination (excluding a few foods at a time from the diet to see whether symptoms are relieved) or by the technique of challenge (initially giving a limited diet to which other foods are gradually added, one at a time, until symptoms appear). If the allergy is mild, it may never be possible to pinpoint the food allergen.

Skin tests are generally of little value in diagnosing food allergies. Also, other conditions in the stomach and intestines that may be quite serious can cause symptoms that mimic food allergy. A careful medical history is the best diagnostic tool.

In some food groups, especially legumes and seafoods, an allergy to one member of the food group may result in being allergic to some other member.

As you can see from the difficulty in diagnosing food allergies, additives—intentional and unintentional, listed and not listed on the label—compound the problem.

Eating anything at a restaurant or fast-food place can be like Russian roulette if you have a severe food allergy, because ingredients are not listed on the menu. You may have to bet your life on the knowledge and honesty of service personnel to tell you what is really in your meal.

Take the case of a young man who had a stuffy nose and recurrent asthma attacks because of allergies. It was known that he was allergic to iodine and peanuts. One day he took his wife out for ice cream at an "old-fashioned ice cream parlor." He ordered a banana split with chocolate and strawberry ice cream. He took a few delicious bites, gasped, grabbed his throat, and turned blue. Without speedy medical attention, he might have died, as did the two young women whose cases were described at the beginning of this chapter. The husband, it turned out, was violently sensitive to artificial chocolate and strawberry flavorings in the "old-fashioned" ice cream.

The young man was a patient of Dr. Stephen Lockey, of Lancaster, Pennsylvania, an allergist who for years had been calling for recognition of allergic reactions to hidden additives. Interviewed for the first edition of *Poisons in Your Food*, Dr. Lockey pointed out that allergy has no respect for age or sex. People of all ages are victims. A few days after birth an infant can develop a skin rash that may last several weeks. Body changes that are probably acquired before birth may set the stage for altered reactions. Colic in infancy can last three months or more and may be the result of sensitization to cow's milk. It can on occasion be caused by breast milk when the mother has drunk cow's milk or some other allergenic substance.

Processed foods, allergy, and children is a topic of great concern to many parents and physicians like Dr. Lockey.

Dr. Howard G. Rapport, writing in the *Journal of Asthma Research,* said:

Allergy is the most important chronic disease of childhood. Allergic illness is responsible for more days of school absence than any other chronic condition. It is the cause of loss of school, play time and growth time. It destroys healthy family life.

The problem of allergic disease in childhood is unfortunately growing more significant each year. The question of what we are able to do about it does not have an easy answer. Every day we are exposed to new types of plastics, synthetic detergents, food additives, insecticides, weed killers and dozens of new chemical compounds which frequently end up in our rivers and reservoirs and the very air we breathe.

Each new compound is, of course, a potential invitation to allergy. New techniques in the production and storage of food have also taken their toll. Permitting and even promoting early weaning and total dependence on manufactured formulas and introduction of solid foods as early as the first or second month of life. Allergically, this has created many problems [as well].[13]

Since the first edition of this book appeared, the FDA has ruled that two common allergenic artificial colorings, FD&C Yellows No. 5 and No. 6, be listed on labels. (Other colorings do not have to be identified.) In the case of the yellows, many people who are sensitive to aspirin are also sensitive to them. Ingestion of the coloring additives can cause facial swelling, swelling of the tissues, stuffy nose, or asthma. As a result, an aspirin-sensitive person who carefully avoids aspirin-containing products might have an asthma attack or serious edema after eating a food containing yellow coloring, and never know why.

SULFITES (SODIUM, POTASSIUM, AND AMMONIUM)

These preservatives, antioxidants, and antibrowning agents used in foods are examples of risk and benefit with all the risk on our side and all the benefit to those who sell us food. There are six sulfiting agents that are currently listed as Generally Recognized as Safe (GRAS) by the FDA. They are sulfur dioxide, sodium sulfite, sodium and potassium bisulfite, and sodium and potassium metabisulfite. The sulfiting agents may be used as preservatives in any food except meat or food that is a recognized source of Vitamin B_1. These agents have been used in many processed foods and in cafeterias and restaurants to prevent fruits, green vegetables, potatoes, and salads from turning brown, as well as to enhance their crispness.

There have been twenty-seven deaths reported associated with sulfites.

Linda Tollefson, DVM, MPH chief, Clinical Nutrition Assessment Section, FDA, says: "Given the limitations of the information available to us, we have determined that 10 of these deaths are probably associated with the use of sulfiting agents, 7 of the deaths are possibly associated with sulfites in either food or drugs, and 10 of the deaths are probably not related to sulfites."[14]

Reactions to sulfites can include acute asthma attacks, loss of consciousness, anaphylactic shock, diarrhea, and nausea occurring soon after ingesting sulfiting agents.

As of April 1, 1989, the FDA had received 976 consumer complaints describing adverse reactions allegedly due to the ingestion of sulfiting agents. Of these, 797 reports were reviewed. The foods most frequently involved were "salad bar," "nonsalad bar fresh fruit and vegetables," "wine," and "seafood."[15]

The FDA banned the use of the preservative on fresh fruits and vegetables and as of this writing is reviewing a proposal to prohibit it on fresh, precut potatoes. The FDA decided in 1988 against extending its ban on the use of sulfites to a variety of foods sold in supermarkets and served in restaurants, including wine, dried fruit, some seafood and condiments. Sulfites must be declared on the labels of wine and packaged foods sold in supermarkets when they are added in excess of 10 ppm (parts per million).

A citizens' petition was submitted by the Center for Science in the Public Interest, Washington, D.C., on October 28, 1982, that asked the FDA to restrict the use of sulfiting agents to a safe residue level in food or require labels on those food products in which sulfiting agents must be used at higher levels to perform essential public health functions.

In the meantime, the California Grape and Tree Fruit League recommended that the Food and Drug Administration rate as Generally Recognized As Safe those sulfiting agents used in sulfur dioxide fumigation within specific limitations and include the use of sulfur dioxide as an ingredient to treat fresh grapes. Stating that the compound is essential to the marketing, transport, storage, and export of table grapes, the group claimed lack of any known substitute for the gaseous compound effective in preventing mold-rot and other storage fungi and in prolonging storage life. A spokesperson for the Wine Institute, which represents 460 domestic wine makers, said that many of the sulfur compounds in wine are natural parts of fermentation, but they are also added to many wines.

The FDA considered requiring the labeling of all sulfite-treated foods used in restaurants, but the FDA felt restaurant labeling would be "labor intensive and difficult to enforce." It would require regular inspection of more than 500,000 eating establishments.[16]

OTHER HIDDEN INGREDIENTS THAT MAY CAUSE AN ALLERGY ATTACK

Did you know some growers, packers, and distributors of yellow variety sweet potatoes artificially color the skins with red dye? We might never have known this except the people who grow the more expensive naturally red sweet potatoes objected.[17]

There are many "hidden" and listed (but often not read) ingredients in foods that may bring on an allergic attack in the sensitive and unsuspecting.

Joseph B. Miller, M.D., a clinical associate professor, department of pediatrics, University of Alabama Medical Center, gathered information about a number of such substances for the sake of his fellow allergists.[18] Among those he identified:

Egg

Egg derivatives are commonly found as labeled or unlabeled ingredients in baking powder, Hollandaise sauce, tartar sauce, some sausages and luncheon meats. Egg is also often used in root beer for producing foam and in coffee and some wines.

Milk

Casein, caseinate, lactose, and whey are derivatives of milk. Most "nondairy creamers" do contain milk products—sodium or calcium caseinate and lactose. Powdered artificial sweeteners often contain lactose (milk).

Soy

Lecithin, food "extenders," and factory-made low-cholesterol food substitutes such as Morningstar Farm® sausages and Betty Crocker Stove Top Stuffing® are derived largely from soy. Soy is in cereals, Lea and Perrins Sauce®, Worcestershire Sauce®, La Choy Soy Sauce®, and La Choy Teriyaki Sauce®. Tuna, sardines, and other foods are often packed in soy oil. Popcorn, potato chips, processed fried fish, and other substances are often fried in soy oil. Soy is the base of many infant formulas.

Cottonseed Oil

Cottonseed oil is in almost all the products listed as containing soybean oil. Cottonseed flour is also used to make gin. Cottonseed is one of the most frequent causes of anaphylactic shock, as described at the beginning of this chapter.

Corn

Corn is found as a hidden ingredient in many foods including dextrose, glucose, dextrin, dextrimaltose, beer, bourbon, Scotch, blended whiskeys, vodka, gin, fortified wines, and many liqueurs. Commercial fructose is now made from corn. Almost all factory-processed sweets contain corn-derived products. So do salami, frankfurters, snack chips, jams, jellies, and most infant formula.

Chocolate

If you have a reaction to chocolate, you should skip cola drinks and karaya gum, often listed on labels as "vegetable gum," because both are from the same botanical family.

Fruits and Vegetables

The pure fruit or vegetable may be fine, according to Dr. Miller, but they are sprayed with insecticides, fungicides, and other chemicals that may bring on an allergic attack. Among the most common coated culprits are peaches, apples, and cherries, which may be sprayed or treated with insecticides ten to fifteen times a season.

Frozen Foods

Frozen fish is often dipped in antibiotics before freezing to retard spoilage. Frozen potatoes are often treated with chemicals such as sodium acid pyrophosphate and sodium EDTA to prevent discoloration. The potatoes are also often coated with methylcellulose to harden when they are fried and produce a crisp outer shell.

Canned and Packaged Foods

Some patients cannot tolerate canned or packaged foods because of the plastic or phenolic resin liner of the inner surface of the can. The soft plastic wrappers used to cover foods have been reported to produce reactions in the sensitive.

CANCER-CAUSING INGREDIENTS

As I mention throughout this book, we are exposed to numerous cancer-causing agents as intentional and unintentional food additives. While allergic or food-sensitivity reactions may occur instantly or over a relatively short period of time, cancer may take decades to develop.

In May 1986, Peter Greenwald, M.D., Dr. P.H. (Doctor of Public Health), director, Division of Cancer Prevention and Control, National Cancer Institute, issued a statement that noted the existence of a general scientific consensus according to which about

80 percent of cancer cases appear to be linked to the way people live their lives. For example, whether or not we smoke, the foods we eat, and certain industrial pollutants all affect our likelihood of getting cancer. "The role of diet in the cause and prevention of cancer is particularly important. In fact, the most comprehensive review to date estimates that 35 percent of cancer deaths may be associated with dietary influences . . ."[19]

The development of cancer is not a simple process. It results from the interaction of the cancer-causing agent with the biological target. The effect is influenced by the susceptibility of your cells, tissues, or organs and your individual immunity. Factors such as age, sex, hormonal status, diet, inheritance, and individual variations in how your body processes chemicals all contribute to your response to a carcinogen: differences as high as a hundredfold or a thousandfold in test animals can be obtained by changing only one factor at a time. Thus valid epidemiological studies are difficult to conduct because reactions to a single carcinogen may not appear in the study groups owing to the varying degrees of susceptibility.

These difficulties are further complicated by the long period—perhaps two to forty years—between exposure to a cancer-causing agent and the development of cancer.

Government agencies maintain that for regulatory purposes they must assume that the results of tests in rodents will closely parallel tumor induction in humans, although they cannot be absolutely certain of this. Therefore, when an agent is a cancer-inducer in animals, mathematical formulas are used to convert a dangerous dosage in human terms. Confirmation, if possible, is based on determining the incidence in humans.

Animal studies do have their limitations. Cancer researchers are particularly concerned about chemicals that may cause 1 case of cancer in about 200,000. Because of cost, most animal studies are limited to 250 to 1,000 animals. In such relatively small samples, a cancer-causing agent that would produce a malignancy in 1 person out of 200,000 would not even show up. Thus, researchers increase dosages until results appear. Once animals in the group develop tumors, statisticians calculate what percentage would contract cancer from a smaller dose.

Imperfect as they are, animal tests do serve as a warning to humans. Had such warnings been heeded, many victims now dead of cancer would be alive today. As early as 1930, for example, scientists reported that exposure to vinyl chloride caused ill effects in laboratory animals. In 1970, Italian scientists noted that rats exposed to high levels of vinyl chloride for one year developed tumors. But it wasn't until 1974, when an alert plant physician at B. F. Goodrich reported three cases of rare liver cancers among workers at a single vinyl-chloride production plant, that the substance was first recognized as a serious cancer threat. Incidentally, vinyl chloride is still permitted by the FDA to be used in coating fresh citrus fruits.[20]

The same tale is told about DES (diethylstilbestrol), the synthetic estrogen. French researchers reported in 1938 that it caused mammary cancer in mice. Similar reports were made during the 1940s and 1950s; yet DES was added to feed and implanted in animals bred for human consumption just to make them weigh more, because producers are paid by the pound. DES was also given to pregnant women to prevent miscarriages. Had observant Massachusetts researchers not noticed rare cancers in young girls and made the correlation between these cancers and the synthetic estrogens taken by their mothers, the tragedy might have continued to escalate.

The FDA had a difficult time getting DES out of the food supply. Cattle and chicken producers kept using it for years; it was still being bootlegged in the early 1980s and may still be today, for all we know.

Detection difficulties posed by the time it takes for cancer to develop are compounded by the mobility of our society: people in our country change jobs, residences, doctors, and hospitals frequently, so that even large-scale adverse health effects from a food additive may go undetected.

Another problem, according to federal investigators, is that epidemiological studies are difficult to conduct because it is seldom possible to separate a single variable from the complex mix of chemical agents to which we are exposed in our work and other environments.

How, then, do you go about proving something is a carcinogen?
Russell Train, former administrator of the Environmental Protection
Agency, said, when ordering the removal of the pesticides heptachlor and chlordane from the market in 1976: *"I have noted some
tendency, not entirely absent from the record, to assert that any
chemical, if fed in sufficiently large amounts, will cause cancer in
test animals. This is not true."* According to Train, a study sponsored by the National Cancer Institute tested 140 pesticides and
industrial chemicals in "two strains of mice and less than 10 percent
of these were found to be carcinogenic." (Heptachlor, as you have
seen on page 19, has not disappeared from the food chain.)

It is, of course, unethical as well as illegal to deliberately test
carcinogens on humans. Therefore, animal experiments must be
used and the data extrapolated to human risks. This does involve
uncertainties.

In many animal experiments the type of cancer produced is
exactly the same as that recorded in human studies. For example,
bladder cancer is produced in man, hamster, dog, and monkey by
2-NA. In other instances species variations result in the induction of
different types of cancer at different locations by the same cancer
agent. Benzidine causes liver-cell carcinoma in the rat and bladder
cancer in man and dog.

The fact that all human carcinogens—with the possible exception
of arsenic—also cause tumors in animals encourages the belief that
these tests are valid. But animal tests are very expensive.

In the early 1970s, Dr. Bruce Ames, then a biochemist at the
University of California at Berkeley, developed a simple test using
common bacteria that reveals whether a chemical is a mutagen. The
test can be done quickly and is relatively inexpensive. Mutagens act
by fouling up the genetic material within a cell. The fact that almost
all of the chemicals known to be carcinogens have also been shown
to be mutagenic in the Ames Test lends credence to the validity of
this test.

In trying to come up with a quick, valid test to identify cancer-
causing agents, Japanese researchers decided to compare the Ames
Test, another laboratory bacteria test (the DNA Repair Test), and a
test that uses the bone marrow of live mice. Dr. M. Hayashi and his

colleagues at Japan's National Institute of Hygienic Sciences studied forty-seven chemicals, including thirty-two synthetic food additives. They tested the chemicals in the bone marrow of eight-week-old male mice.

The Japanese found that twenty-nine out of the thirty-four compounds that were positive in the Ames Test and/or in the chromosomal aberration tests in laboratory dishes were negative in the bone marrow of the mice. The chemicals used in food processing that were positive in *all three* tests were:

- *Chlorine dioxide.* Used as a maturing agent for flour, water-treatment purification, and bleaching fats and oils.
- *Maltol.* A food additive used to impart a "freshly baked flavor to bread and cakes. Used also as a synthetic chocolate, coffee, fruit, maple, nut, and vanilla flavoring agent for beverages, ice cream, ices, candy, baked goods, gelatin desserts, chewing gum, and jelly.
- *Potassium bromate.* A maturing agent and dough conditioner used in flours.
- *Sodium chlorite.* A powerful oxidizer prepared commercially and used to modify food starch up to .5 percent. Used also in water purification.
- *Sodium dehydroacetate.* A preservative used in cut or peeled squash and as a plasticizer, fungicide, and bactericide in some toothpastes.

Since the first edition of *Poisons in Your Food* was published, a number of widely used additives have been removed, after many years of being added to our foods, because they were found to cause cancer or toxicity in animals. Among them are the following:

FOOD COLORINGS
Violet No. 1
Red No. 2
Red No. 3 (Partial ban in 1990)
Red No. 4
Citrus Red No. 2
Orange B

OTHER FOOD ADDITIVES
Borax, a water softener and alkali
Cinnamyl anthranilate, a flavoring
Coumarin, a flavoring
Diethyl pyrocarbonate (DEPC), a growth inhibitor
Diethylstilbestrol (DES), a growth promoter
8-Hydroxyquinoline sulfate, used to aid coagulation in cottage
   cheese.
Monochloracetic acid, a preservative
Nordihydroguaiaretic acid (NDGA), an antioxidant
Oil of sassafras, a flavoring
Safrole, a flavoring, and any oil containing safrole
Thiourea, an antioxidant
Tonka extract, a flavoring

There are other well-known cancer-causing agents identified in
the first edition of *Poisons in Your Food* that are still in our food
today.

NITRATES AND NITRITES

Potassium nitrite is used as a color fixative in the multibillion-
dollar-a-year cured-meat business. Sodium nitrite has the peculiar
ability to react chemically with the myoglobin molecule to impart a
blood-redness to processed meats, to convey tanginess to the palate,
and to resist the growth of *Clostridium botulinum* spores, which can
cause the deadly food poisoning, botulism. The nitrites are used in
cured meats, bacon, bologna, frankfurters, deviled ham, meat
spread, potted meats, spiced ham, Vienna sausages, smoke-cured
tuna fish products, and in smoke-cured shad and salmon.
The problem is that nitrites combine with natural stomach and
food chemicals (secondary amines) to create nitrosamines, among
the most powerful cancer-causing agents known. The U.S. Department of Agriculture, which has jurisdiction over processed meats,
and the FDA, which has jurisdiction over processed poultry, asked
manufacturers to show that the use of nitrites was safe and that
nitrosamines were not formed in the products, as preliminary tests

for bacon showed. Processors claimed there was no alternate chemical substitute for nitrites. They said alternate processing methods could be used but the products would not look or taste the same. Baby-food manufacturers voluntarily removed nitrites from baby foods in the early seventies. The FDA found that adding vitamin C to processed meats prevents or at least retards the formation of nitrosamines.

In 1977, Germany banned nitrites and nitrates except in certain species of fish.

In May 1978, the United States Department of Agriculture announced plans to require bacon manufacturers to reduce their use of nitrites from 150 to 120 ppm and to use preservatives that retard nitrosamine formation. Processors would have been required to keep nitrosamine levels to 10 ppm until an effective substitute for nitrites could be found.

But in August 1978 a new concern about nitrites was raised. The USDA and the FDA issued a joint announcement that the substance has been directly linked to cancer by researchers at the Massachusetts Institute of Technology, Cambridge, and at The Michael Reese Medical Center in Chicago, Illinois, whose studies found very small doses of nitrite or nitrosamines caused cancer in animals. The tumors that developed in mice were similar to human liver tumors and the tumors developed in hamsters were similar to human pancreatic cancer.[21]

However, a committee on nitrite and alternative curing agents in food, formed by the National Research Council, concluded that there was no single agent or process that could replace nitrites completely: "Several chemical and physical treatments appear to be comparable in inhibiting outgrowth of *Clostridium botulinum* spores in types of meat products but none confers the color and flavor that consumers have come to expect in nitrite-cured meats."

In 1980, the FDA revoked its proposed phaseout because manufacturers said there was no adequate substitute for nitrites.

The United States Department of Agriculture's most recent regulations for controlling nitrite levels in bacon allow processors, at their own discretion, to continue to add nitrites at the present levels or use lower levels together with an approved quality control program to prevent spoilage. The process used will determine "how often nitrosamines . . . will be monitored."[22]

Nitrates change into nitrites on exposure to air.

Our major intake of nitrates in foodstuffs comes primarily from vegetables or water supplies that are high in nitrate content. The two most important factors responsible for large accumulations of nitrates in vegetables are the high levels of fertilization with nitrate fertilizers and the tendency of the species to accumulate nitrates.

Nitrates have caused deaths from methemoglobinemia (oxygen cut off to the brain). Because nitrates are difficult to control in processing, they are being used less often. However, they are still employed in long-curing processes, such as for country hams, as well as for dried, cured, and fermented sausages. Again, efforts to ban nitrates have failed because manufacturers claim there is no good substitute for them.

AFLATOXIN

Aflatoxins are produced by molds on peanuts, Brazil nuts, pistachio nuts, almonds, walnuts, pecans, filberts, cottonseed, copra, corn, grain sorghum, millet, and figs. Symptoms of aflatoxin ingestion can be loss of appetite, weight loss, jaundice, cirrhosis, and cancer.

Aflatoxins have been intensively studied since an outbreak of Turkey X disease in England in 1960, when thousands of turkeys died. Investigation showed they died of liver damage and that this liver damage resulted from toxins developed by a mold that grew on the ground nuts (most of which were peanuts) constituting a major portion of their diet.

Aflatoxin B_1 is one of the most potent liver-cancer-causing agents known.[23] In experiments, low levels of Aflatoxin B_1—as low as 1 ppb (part per billion)—fed continuously in the diet produced cancer in 100 percent of the rats tested. A relatively large dose—five milligrams—given just once also caused cancer in rats. In the northwestern part of the United States, rainbow trout died of liver cancer developed, it was believed, from aflatoxin-contaminated wheat, but there was no evidence of a relationship between the outbreak and human cancer.

In addition to liver cancer, aflatoxins have been implicated in the formation of tumors of the stomach, kidney, and other tissues in animals.

The effect on humans of aflatoxins has been difficult to demonstrate: since moldy food is not aesthetically pleasing for human consumption, it often ends up in animal feed (milk currently on the market contains aflatoxins because cows are sometimes fed moldy grain).

Researchers have suspected the presence of some common substance in the outbreak of liver cancer in certain geographic areas. In some parts of Africa and China, where there is a high incidence of liver cancer, aflatoxin contamination is common.

The FDA has had informal standards for peanut aflatoxin for a decade. Similar regulations are planned for other affected commodities.

There is no known way to remove the mold once it occurs in meal. Peanut oils, however, seem to be free of mold because of the alkaline treatment they receive during processing. When a batch of peanuts is imported containing aflatoxin levels that are too high for us to eat, the current method of control is to dilute the contaminated batch with a clean batch to bring the level down to acceptable proportions.[24]

Aflatoxins have been detected in trace quantities in certain batches of peanut butter.[25]

The drought of 1988–89 caused the FDA to worry about aflatoxins in milk and they alerted state health officials to look for the contamination. When inspectors did find some milk with 0.5 ppb or more of aflatoxin, the milk was dumped.[26]

In 1988, the FDA found that about 6 percent of field corn in areas with known or potential problems contained more than 20 ppb of aflatoxin, the limit for grain intended for direct human consumption. But in a test of finished, ready-to-eat cereal and chips, the FDA found no aflatoxin. About 2 percent of corn flour and cornmeal, however, was found to be above 20 ppb in the FDA's tests. Although the agency's policy is to remove such products from the market, the FDA says that the amount of aflatoxin would be greatly reduced by cooking the grits, corn flour, or cornmeal.[27]

The FDA permits corn with higher aflatoxin levels to be used for nondairy animals, such as beef cattle and poultry. According to the FDA, their studies have shown that such FDA-approved levels have not harmed the animals and have not resulted in significant amounts of aflatoxin in meat or eggs.[28]

ARTIFICIAL SWEETENERS

Most Americans are more worried about how much they weigh than about the purity of their food. When the United States secretary of health, education, and welfare restricted the use of the artificial sweetener cyclamate on October 18, 1969, more than 175 million Americans, including young children, were ingesting the chemical. The rise in the use of cyclamate, which was intended originally only for diabetics and others on sugar-restricted, medically supervised diets, was from 0.25 million pounds in 1955 to more than 17 million pounds in 1969. Sixty-nine percent of the artificial sweetener was used in beverages, 19 percent in table sweeteners, 6 percent in foods, 4 percent in nonfood items, and 2 percent was exported.[29]

Cyclamates were first marketed in the early 1950s, for use in diet foods. In 1958, they were placed on the Generally Recognized As Safe list, so that no restrictions were imposed on their use. As early as 1962, scientists began to have doubts about the unrestrained intake of cyclamates. In the fall of 1964, the *Medical Letter*, published by a group of prominent American physicians, asserted that excessive use of these sweeteners was against the public interest.

In 1965, the Wisconsin Alumni Research Foundation reported that after a diet of 5 percent calcium cyclamate for nine months and 95 percent normal nutrition, laboratory rats grew 12 percent less than did a control group not receiving the sweetener. When the diet was changed to include 10 percent cyclamate, the rats suffered a growth impairment of 50 percent.

In 1966, FDA researchers studied the sweeteners after Japanese scientists said that birth defects associated with artificial sweeteners had been found in experimental animals. The National Academy of Sciences announced that the new study was "appropriate in the light of the new toxicological information on the increased use of artificial sweeteners."

Research at Albany, New York, had already shown that cyclamates cause symptoms imitating hyperthyroidism, which resulted in patients being treated for the hormone disorder erroneously. Furthermore, the Albany researchers found that some people convert cyclamates into cyclohexylamine (CHA), a substance that raises blood pressure.[30]

On June 5, 1969, scientists at the University of Wisconsin reported to Abbott Laboratories, manufacturer of cyclamates and sponsor of the research, that a significant incidence of bladder tumors had been found in white Swiss mice in two experiments in which pellets of cholesterol and cyclamates had been implanted into the lumen of the urinary bladder. Representatives of Abbott Laboratories discussed the matter with representatives of the National Cancer Institute and the Food and Drug Administration, and they came to the conclusion that the cancer-causing properties of the pellet did not convict cyclamates that were given orally, but that further studies should be performed.[31]

On October 8, 1969, an Abbott scientist, conducting experiments at the Food and Drug Research Laboratories in Long Island, New York, noticed that there appeared to be bladder lesions in rats fed a 10:1 mixture of cyclamate sodium/saccharin sodium over a two-year period. During this study, many of these rats were also shown to be able to convert cyclamate to cyclohexylamine.[32]

On October 13, representatives of Abbott Laboratories met with FDA researchers to review the study of cyclamate sodium/saccharin sodium mixture. Of 240 rats, 7 males and 1 female showed bladder tumors rarely seen in rats.

On October 18, HEW Secretary Robert H. Finch ordered the artificial sweetener cyclamate removed from the Generally Recognized As Safe list.[33]

Further confirming evidence of the cyclamates' cancer-inducing properties developed, and new evidence showed the chemical's ability to cause genetic defects and birth defects in chick embryos.[34]

After the ban, the FDA banished to the boondocks Dr. Howard L. Richardson, its chief pathologist, who had made public a 1950 agency study on the questionable safety of cyclamates. The 1950 experiment showed the same cancer dangers that led to its ban by the government in 1969.[35]

More than twenty years later, there is a great deal of pressure to bring cyclamates back. Researchers say that the bladder tumors associated with cyclamates in the experiments were really caused by irritation from the cholesterol pellets that contained it. They say that saccharin, the artificial sweetener substituted for cyclamates in most artificially sweetened products, is a tumor promoter and more potentially harmful than cyclamates.[36] Discovered in 1879, saccharin is pound for pound about three hundred times as sweet as natural sugar. Cyclamates have about thirty times the sweetness of sugar but were preferred to the older saccharin because they did not have saccharin's characteristic bitter aftertaste.

Saccharin was used along with cyclamates in the experiments that led to the ban on cyclamates. Dr. George T. Bryan, the same researcher who conducted the experiments at the University of Wisconsin, has charged that saccharin causes more dangerous tumors in mice than do cyclamates, and should be banned.[37]

The FDA asked that the National Research Council of the National Academy of Sciences review material available concerning the safety of saccharin. The preliminary report by NAS-NRC said that there is no immediate danger and that saccharin should be studied further. Government studies then showed that saccharin was indeed a weak carcinogen or tumor promoter—it didn't cause cancer by itself but helped other carcinogens to do the job. But the public outcry prevented the removal of the sweetener from the market. The saccharin issue is in limbo as of this writing.

Americans are still overweight, despite their use of artificial sweeteners. More than 15 percent of the men and 20 percent of the women in the United States between the ages of twenty-five and forty-four are obese, and the rate has been increasing by about 1 percent per year.[38]

It is doubtful that a newer and more popular sweetener, aspartame, will have any more effect on weight loss than has saccharin or cyclamates. And there are also serious questions about aspartame's safety. The questions are not related to cancer but to how aspartame may affect the brain and nerves.

Aspartame

Aspartame (NutraSweet®) is produced commercially from two amino acids, L-phenylalanine and L-aspartic acid. It is one hundred to two hundred times sweeter than sugar. The FDA approved it in 1974 but objections based on the possibility that aspartame could cause brain damage led to a stay, or legal postponement, of that approval. An FDA investigation of records of animal studies that were conducted for Searle drug and aspartame approvals raised additional questions. The FDA arranged for an independent audit, which took more than two years and concluded that the aspartame studies and results were authentic. The agency then organized an expert board of inquiry, whose members concluded that the evidence did not support the charge that aspartame might kill clusters of brain cells or cause other damage. However, persons with an inborn error of metabolism, phenylketonuria, must avoid protein foods such as meat that contain phenylalanine—one of the two components of aspartame. The board did, however, recommend that aspartame not be approved until further long-term animal testing could be conducted to rule out the possibility that aspartame might cause brain tumors. The FDA's Bureau of Foods viewed the study data then available and concluded that the board's concern was unfounded. Aspartame was approved for use as a tabletop sweetener in certain dry foods in 1981 and in soft drinks two years later.

In 1984, news reports, fueled by the announcement that the Arizona Department of Health Services was testing soft drinks containing aspartame to see if it deteriorated into toxic levels of methyl alcohol under storage conditions, created alarm. The Arizona health department acted after the director of the Food Sciences and Research Laboratory at Arizona State University submitted a study alleging that higher than normal temperatures could lead to a dangerous breakdown in the chemical composition of aspartame.[39] The authors checked with representatives of the FDA, who said there were higher levels of methyl alcohol in regular fruit juices, and so as far as the agency was concerned, fears about decomposition were unfounded.

As of April 1989, the FDA had received 4,398 consumer complaints describing adverse reactions to aspartame.[40] By far the most common complaint was "headache," followed by "dizziness or problems with balance," "change in mood quality," "vomiting and nausea," and "abdominal pain and cramps," in descending order. There were also changes in vision, fatigue and weakness, memory loss, sleep problems, and changes in menstrual pattern among the complaints. There were 239 seizures and convulsions reported.[41]

Richard Wurtman, M.D., a professor of neuroendocrine regulation at MIT, who has conducted laboratory studies on aspartame, says that there are several groups of people who might be especially susceptible to high doses of phenylalanine. These include people who are taking drugs that act on the brain (such as medications for high blood pressure), people with a history of seizures, youngsters, and pregnant women. Dr. Wurtman suggests that moderate amounts of aspartame a day should not be hazardous for adults who do not fall into these categories.[42]

Approximately 40 percent of the consumers reporting an adverse reaction associated with an aspartame-containing product mentioned diet soft drinks as the source of exposure, and 20 percent mentioned tabletop sweeteners. Puddings and gelatins, lemonade, Kool-Aid®, hot chocolate, iced tea, and chewing gum followed in descending order.[43]

Since this artificial sweetener is not vital to one's well-being—except perhaps for some diabetics who have sweets cravings—you should ask yourself if it is really a necessity in your diet, especially since the second major ingredient, glutamate, is being intensively studied as a neurotoxin involved in brain degeneration, particularly Alzheimer's disease.

Researchers at Albert Einstein College of Medicine in New York City, collaborating with Indian and Israeli scientists, have been working with a substance isolated from chick-peas that causes nerve damage similar to that caused by amyotrophic lateral sclerosis (ALS), Lou Gehrig's disease. The toxic component, BOAA, is chemically related to two approved food additives—aspartame and glutamate.[44]

GLUTAMATE, MSG, AND YOUR BRAIN

Glutamate, a salt of the amino acid glutamic acid, is a remarkably potent, rapidly acting nerve toxin in laboratory cell cultures. It causes swelling of a nerve after only ninety seconds of contact.

Why glutamate causes nerve injury is unknown. More than a decade ago it was believed that glutamate neurotoxicity is a direct consequence of overexciting the nerves. More recently it has been thought that a calcium influx triggered by glutamate exposure may be involved in glutamate toxicity. Under normal circumstances, the brain appears well equipped to handle large amounts of glutamate in a harmless fashion, rapidly removing it and sequestering it inside cells, where it is nontoxic. In recent years, however, a number of disease states have been linked to glutamate neurotoxicity—among them, Huntington's disease, a hereditary brain-degenerating condition, and nerve loss associated with acute brain or spinal cord injury due to stroke or trauma, where injured nervous tissue may be unable to safely absorb glutamate and may, in addition, release glutamate from storage, leading to extension of the original injury.

It is now suspected that glutamate and related neurotransmitters may also be involved in the nerve tangles that form the brain cell degeneration found in Alzheimer's disease victims. Some researchers have demonstrated that in Alzheimer's disease there is a decrease in the number of brain receptors to which glutamate binds.

The cause of tangled nerve formations in Alzheimer's is still not understood, but the fact that such tangles are in the brain cells involved with processing glutamate raises interesting questions. Why are glutamate nerve cells susceptible to tangle formations? Is it a genetic abnormality or do viruses invade this particular cell type? Both possibilities are intriguing. What if these neurons are producing abnormally high levels of glutamate, which might then act as a toxin? If this is the case, the nerve degeneration associated with Alzheimer's disease might be halted with drugs that inhibit the effects of excess glutamate.[45]

Not only are we swallowing glutamate in aspartame, we may be sprinkling it on food in the form of MSG, monosodium glutamate, used commercially to intensify spice flavorings in meats, condiments, pickles, soups, candies, and baked goods. It is also in products listed as "hydrolyzed vegetable protein."

Researchers believe that the so-called Chinese restaurant syndrome is caused by a sudden elevation of glutamate in the blood, which produces a blood vessel response.[46] MSG has been found to cause brain damage in young rodents and brain-damage effects in rabbits, chicks, and monkeys. Baby-food processors removed MSG from products voluntarily. It is on the FDA's list of additives whose mutagenic, teratogenic, subacute, and reproductive effects need further study. In 1980, the final report to the FDA from the Select Committee on Generally Recognized As Safe Substances stated that while no evidence in the available information about MSG demonstrates a hazard to the public at current-use levels, the uncertainties that exist require that additional studies be conducted. GRAS status continues while tests are being completed and evaluated.

MSG is an unnecessary addition to food and therefore is not worth even the slightest risk!

There is new evidence that brain damage is caused by natural food ingredients closely related to glutamate and aspartame, according to John Olney, M.D., a psychiatrist at Washington University in St. Louis: "Twenty years ago, glutamate was shown to cause brain damage in infant animals and the Food and Drug Administration did nothing to restrict its use. Since then, it has become increasingly evident that glutamate and closely related substances are neurotoxins that can cause human neurodegenerative diseases."[47] Dr. Olney said that not only may glutamate and aspartate cause degenerative nerve damage in adults, but that "accumulating evidence has abundantly confirmed earlier studies showing that the immature brain is much more vulnerable than the adult brain to the toxic actions of glutamate and aspartate. It might be advisable for the FDA to quit sanctioning the unrestricted use of these excitotoxins in foods fed to young children and to begin educating mothers against feeding excitotoxins to children."[48]

Glutamate, in the form of MSG, is the world's most widely used food additive; aspartate comprises half of the aspartame (Nutrasweet®) molecule and is rapidly becoming equally pervasive.

Dr. Olney pointed out that natural foods containing glutamate-like substances can cause serious neurological disorders. He described an episode of food poisoning that occurred in December, 1987, involving more than 150 people in Canada who ate mussels. The poisoning caused acute destruction of nerve cells among the four Canadians who died and permanent brain damage with symptoms similar to Alzheimer's disease in twelve of the survivors. An analysis found the mussels to be high in domoic acid, an excitotoxic-chemical relative of glutamate.

NEUROTOXINS

The possibility that food additives such as MSG and aspartame are potential neurotoxins—substances damaging to the brain and nerves—was not considered in the first edition of this book. Even today, no testing for neurotoxicity is required, although some researchers believe that neurotoxic food additives are a greater threat than are cancer-causing agents.

Alzheimer's disease now affects 2.5 million people in the United States. Its course is marked by a gradual loss of memory, ability to communicate and, eventually, physical capabilities.

In addition to the reports about glutamate and aspartame, it has been noted that there is a buildup of aluminum and fluoride in the brains Alzheimer's patients.[49] Some argue that the buildup of aluminum—which is in a number of food additives—is a result rather than a cause of the brain condition. The same, they say, holds true for fluoride, which of course is added to water and toothpaste to prevent tooth decay. Are they right? Could aluminum in food and water speed the downward course of Alzheimer's?

The aluminum additives currently added to food are:

• *Alum.* Used in food packaging and used to harden gelatins.
• *Aluminum ammonium sulfate.* Used to purify drinking water; used in baking powder; used as a buffering and neutralizing agent in milling and in the cereal industry.
• *Aluminum calcium sulfate.* Anticaking agent used in table salt and vanilla powder.
• *Aluminum hydroxide.* An alkali used as a leavening agent in baked goods.

- *Aluminum nicotinate.* Used as a source of niacin in special diet foods.
- *Aluminum oleate.* Used in food packaging.
- *Aluminum palmitate.* Used in packaging.
- *Aluminum phosphide.* Used to fumigate processed foods.
- *Aluminum potassium sulfate (potash alum; potassium alum).* Used as a firming agent in sugar processing and as a carrier for bleaching agents; used in the production of sweet pickles, cereal, flours, bleached flours, and cheese.
- *Aluminum sodium sulfate.* A firming agent and carrier for bleaching agents.
- *Aluminum stearate.* Used in chewing-gum bases; used as a defoaming agent in beet-sugar and yeast processing.
- *Aluminum sulfate (cake alum; patent alum).* A firming agent used in processing sweet and dill pickles and as a modifier for food starch.
- *Sodium silico aluminate.* An anticaking agent used in table salt (up to 2 percent), in dried egg yolks (up to 2 percent), in sugar (up to 1 percent), and in baking powder (up to 5 percent).

While aluminum is suspect when it appears in the brains of the elderly, there are a number of food additives suspected of affecting the brains of the young.

Attention Deficit Disorder (With Hyperactivity) consists of hyperactivity, impulsivity, distractibility, and excitability.[50] Hyperactivity essentially is a description of the child's basic personality. It may be a temporary state of anxiety or a subclinical seizure disorder, or it may reflect a true hyperkinetic state. The syndrome also may be strictly "in the eyes of the beholder." In one study of teacher ratings, older teachers rated more children hyperactive than did younger teachers.

The extent of the syndrome is not clear, but it has been estimated that it involves between 5 and 10 percent of American schoolchildren. The cluster of symptoms does not represent a single disease. Rather than have a single etiology, the syndrome may be secondary to:

1. Organic factors such as trauma, infection, lead intoxication, and significant hypoxia.

2. Genetically defined predisposing factors.

3. Psychosocial factors such as anxiety, maternal depression, and environmental stress.

In some children the cause is unclear. The possible relationship between Attention Deficit Disorder (With Hyperactivity) and natural salicylates as well as other food additives was presented by Dr. Benjamin Feingold in 1973. Aspirin is a salicylate. On the basis of experience concerning treatment of an adult patient who had aspirin intolerance, Feingold promoted a theory that hyperactive behavior and learning disorders in children might be the result of a reaction to natural salicylates in certain foods. Later, because of the known cross-reactivity between aspirin and tartrazine (FD&C Yellow No. 5), all colors were suspected of being offenders; still later, the preservatives sodium benzoate and BHA/BHT (butylated hydroxyanisole/butylated hydroxytoluene) were suspected. A regimen called the Kaiser-Permanente Diet (K-P Diet or Feingold Diet) was popularized by Feingold in a book on the subject. The special diet, devoid of foods suspected of having not only significant levels of natural salicylates but also colors and preservatives, was alleged to produce improvement in 50 percent of the patients who had the Attention Deficit Syndrome (With Hyperactivity).

The Feingold hypothesis found some support, and several clinical studies were set up to evaluate the theory. Investigation focused on the role of food colors in this hypothesis. Reviews of these studies have led to the following impressions, which are amplified in the published proceedings of the Consensus Development Conference on Defined Diets and Childhood Hyperactivity, held at the National Institutes of Health in January 1982:

1. The Feingold type of diet *may* be helpful for a *small* number of young children with hyperkinesis (not 50 percent, as Feingold stated); however, these decreases in hyperactivity were not observed consistently.

2. In susceptible children challenge with very high doses of food colors might produce a pharmacologic-like effect to depress learning in a specific test situation.

3. Allergic (hypersensitivity) as well as other immunologic reactions to foods or food additives probably have nothing to do with any observed effects of the diet on behavior.

Only the FD&C Red Dye No. 3 (erythrosine) has been shown in the laboratory to inhibit dopamine, the brain chemical involved in movement. This is thought by some to offer an explanation of the effects of certain foods on childhood behavior. FD&C Red Dye No. 3 was partially removed from use in food in 1990 because it caused thyroid cancer in rats. It was banned for use in cake frostings, cheese rinds, and in some processed fruits and juices, but only for new products. Those products with FD&C Red No. 3 already on the market can continue to be sold.[51]

Sugar as an additive—one that is pushed to children in all sorts of advertisements in cereal and candy—is another suspect in brain-behavior problems.[52]

BABY FOOD

In 1969, I pointed out that baby food contained sodium nitrite and high amounts of salt and sugar as well as monosodium glutamate and modified starches. Still another additive to which children may be exposed in ice cream, jellies, chocolate drinks, icings, and certain candies is carboxymethyl cellulose. Made from a cotton byproduct, it is added to these foods as a stabilizer. On the super-market shelves, I found it in every one of the highly advertised mixes children are encouraged to put in their milk. Carboxymethyl cellulose has been shown to cause cancer in animals.[53]

Baby-food producers are extremely responsive to any perception of harm parents may suspect in their products. I am happy to write that baby-food companies voluntarily have removed the nitrites and salt since 1969.

Starches, modified to make them more easily digestible, are still in there. Questions about safety have arisen because babies do not have the resistance of adults to chemicals. Among chemicals used to modify starch are propylene oxide, succinic anhydride, aluminum sulfate, and sodium hydroxide. Modified starch has been on the FDA's top priority list for reevaluation since 1980, but nothing new has been reported about it by the agency since then.[54]

The baby-food manufacturers made changes despite the pontificating of Fredrick J. Stare, M.D., professor of nutrition and head of the department of nutrition at Harvard School of Public Health, and Dr. Charles A. Janeway, professor of pediatrics at Harvard Medical School, who together wrote an indignant article, "Are All Baby Foods Special Dietary Foods?", that appeared in the prestigious *New England Journal of Medicine* on September 7, 1967. Doctors Stare and Janeway referred to the Food and Drug Administration's pending revision of regulations for food of special use.

We are disturbed . . . by the interpretation that may be given those responsible for the enforcement to the definition of Special Dietary Foods that would place ordinary baby foods in this classification.

There are few cases in which infant tolerances for certain food additives—for example, calcium silicate—are considered to be lower than adult tolerance. These differences do not appear to be valid reasons for classifying all baby foods as special dietary foods, particularly since these situations have been handled quite satisfactorily by the setting of specific tolerances for their use in baby foods under the food additive regulations.

Those whom we have consulted in the "baby food" industry contend that the reclassification of baby foods as special dietary-purpose foods would work a hardship on current business practices and serve no advantage to the consumer. Reclassification would probably make necessary certain changes in labeling (for example, it would be necessary to note the source of all ingredients and to specify all flavoring ingredients by their generic names). This would add more copy to labels that are already too small to be read with ease.

As a mother of allergic children, I was certainly distressed that a nutritionist of international renown and a respected pediatrician could make that last statement. Certainly everything that is put into baby-food jars should be described on the label. If necessary, make a bigger label or even a bigger jar. Labeling is not foolproof, however. In 1988, two of Beech-Nut Nutrition Corporation's executives were found guilty of more than eight hundred violations of federal law in the manufacture and sale of millions of containers of sugar, water, and flavoring marketed as "100 percent" apple juice.[55]

As for baby foods being under a special dietary protection, the following month a government official answered the article in the *New England Journal of Medicine* by pointing out that strained and chopped fruits and vegetables marketed as foods for infants are, in fact, classified as foods for special dietary use and have been since 1941.

CHEMICALS IN COMBINATION

In the first edition of *Poisons in Your Food,* I described the "epidemic" among apparently healthy Canadian, American, and Belgian men in their midforties who suddenly dropped dead. The only thing they had in common was a love of drinking beer. Autopsies showed that the heart muscle of the beer drinkers had been destroyed in a peculiar way.[56]

It was determined that cobalt, added to beer to improve the quality of the foam, was at fault. It was also determined that neither beer nor cobalt alone caused the destruction; the chemicals had to work in tandem.

One of the dangers that are becoming more and more a matter of concern among eminent scientists is the effects of chemicals that may be harmless alone but in combination may be extremely toxic. Such chemical interaction in food has been dramatically demonstrated by the more than thirty-one cases of the "depressed cheese eaters." After taking Parnate, a medicine that combats mental depression, and then eating cheese, these people suffered severe high blood pressure that resulted in symptoms ranging from convulsions to strokes. Parnate inhibits the brain chemical monoamine oxidase (MAO). Cheese and other foods, such as beers, wines, yogurt, and beans, contain the natural chemical tyramine. Together, Parnate and tyramine combine to explode the blood pressure.

The fact is that no one knows how the sixty-three thousand chemicals in common use today interact in our bodies. The *Journal of Food Science* carried a report in 1976 about a small-scale attempt to determine the extent of the problem. When three additives were tested one at a time on rats, the animals stayed well. When the additives were tested two at a time, the rats became ill, and when all three were tested at the same time, all the animals died within fourteen days.

WHAT YOU CAN DO TO LOWER YOUR RISKS OF CANCER AND NEUROTOXICITY

- Learn the ingredients to avoid, and read package labels.
- Eat fewer processed foods—the more chemicals added, the higher the risk.
- Do not buy products with aluminum additives listed on the label.
- Skip monosodium glutamate. It is a completely unnecessary additive.
- Cut down on salt.
- If you must take artificial sweeteners, do so in moderation and do not give them to your children or your aging parents.
- If you must eat nitrite-laced meats, include at the same time a food or drink high in vitamin C—for example, orange juice, grapefruit juice, cranberry juice, or lettuce.
- Make sure the nuts you eat are fresh.
- Keep peanut butter and nuts in the refrigerator to cut down the formation of mold.
- Avoid lead-soldered cans. They are usually made by crimping or overlapping the edges of the seam and filling the joint with solder. That's why leaded seams tend to be messy. Lead-free soldering can generally have either no seam or a smooth one. If you run your finger down the seam and feel unevenness through the label, odds are that lead solder has been used.
- It's a good idea to remove food from cans as soon as you open them. Tests have shown that the lead content of acidic foods— like fruit juices and tomatoes—increases when they are stored in open leaded cans.

4 ⌐ Meat and Poultry Hazards

My daughter had a case of hives, those itchy welts that arise from an allergy. The pediatrician could not find the source of the problem, so he sent us to an allergist, who was equally puzzled. Finally, the allergist—after tracking down every other possibility to no avail—said, "Maybe it is the penicillin in the milk."

"What's penicillin doing in the milk?" I asked, not only as a mother but as a newspaper science editor.

"Well," the allergist said, "antibiotics are put in animal feed and farmers treat cows for mastitis [an udder infection] with penicillin. They don't need a prescription to use antibiotics on farm animals."

On investigating the situation, I discovered that farmers were supposed to throw away the milk of penicillin-treated cows for several days after the treatment ceased. However, farmers pool milk, so it is difficult to determine who put the penicillin in the pool.

I found that yogurt companies have their own milk supplies because milk from outside dairies often contains antibiotics that kill the yogurt culture.

My discovery that milk may contain traces of antibiotics evolved into the first edition of this book. I assumed, as you probably did, that all our milk and food is carefully inspected by government agencies before it gets to our dinner tables. That was not so then and it is not so now.

Since 1950, antibiotics have been widely used to stimulate the growth of young chickens, cattle, and pigs. It was discovered that adding low levels of antibiotics to animal feed improved their weight gain by 10 to 11 percent. The medications are also used to increase egg production. Antibiotics are administered at higher levels in feed or drinking water or by injection in the treatment of various diseases of livestock. In fact, almost 50 percent of the antibiotics used in the United States are used for animals.[1]

There are 750 drug products approved for use in food animals. About 30 percent of chickens, 80 percent of veal calves and pigs, and 60 percent of the beef raised for food in the United States are routinely given medicated feed.[2]

Antibiotics approved today by the FDA for growth promotion in animals are: bacitracin, bambemycins, chlortetracycline, erythromycin, lincomycin, monensin, oleandomycin, oxytetracycline, tylosin and virginiamycin.[3]

Penicillin is being added to the feed and drinking water of salmon, catfish, lobsters, chicken, swine, and turkeys.[4]

Penicillin is widely used to treat mastitis, which at any given time affects more than 25 percent of the 26 million cattle in the United States. Ironically, although antibiotic treatment has been shown to eliminate one kind of mastitis, it is frequently replaced by another kind of infection.[5]

The FDA is now trying to control the dispensing of prescription veterinary drugs by issuing them only to veterinarians, although it is a difficult job with shortages of personnel and money to monitor the situation.

Can penicillin used to treat sick cows or added to animal feed affect the users of dairy products? Two cases of a Whittier, California, physician, Dr. Murray C. Zimmerman, answered that question.[6]

A young man who had an injection of penicillin developed severe hives, arthritis, and fever. For sixty days, his symptoms were partially suppressed by massive doses of steroid drugs, antihistamines, epinephrine, calcium, and various other medications. He continued to have hives for nine weeks, until he was given Neutrapen, a drug that neutralizes penicillin. His symptoms cleared up almost completely within forty-eight hours.

However, every time he ate dairy products, he had mild, repeated attacks of his symptoms. At the request of Dr. Zimmerman and another physician, the patient ate dairy products in their presence, and the hives soon followed. As little as eight ounces of milk brought on the attack.

If the patient was given Neutrapen in advance, he was able to eat dairy products without symptoms. One time, the doctors gave the patient an injection of plain salt water, which he thought was Neutrapen. Upon eating dairy products, the patient again had the hives, confirming the presence of penicillin allergy connected with dairy products.

Another of Dr. Zimmerman's patients, a thirty-five-year-old woman, received a penicillin injection for an industrial injury. She had hives, although she had no previous allergic history. She was given Neutrapen and her hives cleared. She was told to avoid dairy products. A short time later, she had a severe outbreak of hives but denied all penicillin exposure. She finally admitted eating Roquefort cheese three hours before the hives began, saying: "I didn't think you could find out so easily that I cheated a little bit."

Researchers from the State University of New York at Buffalo reported the case of a woman who drank a glass of milk and suddenly developed generalized itching, a rash, and a severe headache. She had purchased the milk from a supermarket, which in turn had purchased it from a commercial dairy. The dairy reported that the milk was purchased from numerous local farmers, and a routine check for penicillin content was made about twice a month. When the State University researchers tested the bottle of milk they found approximately 10 units of penicillin per milliliter.[7]

Traces of one antibiotic in your food can make you allergic to other antibiotics given to you for medical purposes. Bacitracin, for example, which is used to promote growth in animal feed, can cause an allergic cross-reaction in humans that may prevent the effective use of kanamycin, neomycin, streptomycin, and pardomonomycin for the treatment of infections.[8]

Only a certain percentage of the population may be allergic to antibiotics and thus be affected by traces of them hidden in food, but the entire population can be affected by another side effect of antibiotic residues.

In the first edition of *Poisons in Your Food,* experts warned that the lacing of animal feed with antibiotics and the subsequent residue in the meat we eat would result in antibiotic-resistant bacteria. Thus, a necessary antibiotic may be ineffective when used to treat an infection in humans.

This warning has come true. Meat and poultry and humans have become infected with antibiotic-resistant strains of bacteria.

Tetracycline, used to treat calves, sheep, swine, chickens, and turkeys, is also used to treat foodborne illnesses in humans such as *Yersinia pestis, Brucella, Escherichia coli,* and *Shigella* (see chapter 6). In the *Physicians Desk Reference,* which doctors use to find information about the drugs they prescribe, there is a caution about tetracycline: "As with other antibiotics, use of this drug may result in overgrowth of *nonsusceptible* organism including fungi. It may also cause hypersensitive reactions such as hives, swelling, anaphylaxis, tachycardia [irregular heart beat] and exacerbation of lupus erythematosus."

The FDA in 1968 proposed revoking the residue tolerance of chlortetracycline and oxytetracycline in fish and poultry. Today chlortetracycline is cleared for application to raw poultry, fish, scallops, and shrimps to retard spoilage, with a tolerance of 7 ppm (parts per million) for uncooked poultry and one of 5 ppm for raw marine products. They are still being widely used with the FDA's approval.

Certain antibiotics of the tetracycline class have also been found to strain baby teeth and cause sensitivity to light, skin rash, and liver toxicity as well as interference with kidney function.[9]

The residue tolerances for tetracyclines in raw poultry and fish were established on the theory that residue in poultry would be destroyed in cooking and residue in raw seafood would not constitute a danger. However, after years of use, it was discovered this is not the case.

Nitrofurans are used extensively in chickens and turkeys and to a lesser extent in swine. Of the two nitrofurans still approved for use in feeds, furazolidone is the most widely used. It and, to a lesser extent, nitrofurazone are used in poultry and swine for growth promotion, feed efficiency, disease prevention, and disease treatment. The government was advised to stop using nitrofurans as far back as 1979.[10] According to the *Physicians Desk Reference,* some strains of intestinal bacteria are now resistant to nitrofurans taken as medication primarily to treat urinary tract infections. Furthermore, allergic reactions and lung side effects are not uncommon.[11]

The British curbed antibiotics in feed in 1969 after studies in Britain found possible hazards to human health. In May 1970, then FDA Commissioner Charles C. Edwards, M.D., appointed an eleven-member committee to study the use of antibiotics in animal feed and medication. Nothing happened to change the status quo.

In 1989, according to a "new risks" assessment made for the FDA by the National Academy of Science's Institute of Medicine (IOM), the group "was unable to find data directly implicating subtherapeutic doses of antibiotics in livestock with illnesses in people" or to come up with a "numerical answer" about the risk of animal medication posed to humans.[12] The IOM estimated that the doses of antibiotics given to livestock to promote growth or prevent infection would account for less than 2 percent of the human deaths due to foodborne, antibiotic-resistant *Salmonella.* (Although officially only somewhere between 150 and 220 deaths are known to be caused by *Salmonella* each year, the IOM estimates that because of underreporting, the actual figure may be closer to 500.)

The committee felt that stopping the use of antibiotics to promote growth in livestock might reduce the total number of human deaths due to *Salmonella* poisoning, but that such results could not be supported scientifically.

One has to wonder how much one government agency talks to another—or listens. Dr. Mitchell Cohen, a bacterial disease expert at the Centers for Disease Control, says that the percentage of *Salmonella* resistant to antibiotics is increasing. He estimates that between 20 and 30 percent of all cases of *Salmonella* infections involve bacteria that are resistant to antibiotics.[13] (*Salmonella* is just one of two thousand closely related bacteria, all of which cause diarrhea, vomiting, and fever.)

"This threatens treatment," he adds. "While most cases of salmonella infections do not require antibiotics, the drugs are needed when the bacteria cause meningitis [inflammation of the brain covering] or infections of the bloodstream. As the frequency of resistance to these antibiotics increases, the physician is left with fewer drugs to use."

Physicians from the Centers for Disease Control in Atlanta and the Los Angeles County Department of Health reported that they had tracked a California outbreak of antibiotic-resistant *Salmonella* in forty-five victims to undercooked meat. The meat was then tracked to the slaughterhouse and from there to the dairy farms where the cattle were routinely treated with small doses of antibiotics.

Publishing their findings in the *New England Journal of Medicine,* in March 1987, the researchers also indicated that the creation of antibiotic-resistant *Salmonella* is probably a much greater problem than was previously thought.[14]

The California outbreak occurred when dairy cattle that were routinely fed a number of different antibiotics developed *Salmonella* infections that could not easily be treated. The cattle were sold to slaughterhouses and meat packers and eventually turned into hamburger.[15] The bacteria were carried along at each step in the process and caused infections when undercooked hamburgers were sold in fast-food restaurants or prepared at home from meat sold in supermarkets, the study reported.

Another disturbing example of antibiotics found in animal feed involves sulfa drugs used in chicken, turkey, swine, and cattle feed for growth promotion and disease prevention.

In 1988, the *FDA Consumer* noted that a widely used wine and cattle drug, sulfamethazine, was undergoing a safety review.[16] "A study by the National Center for Toxicological Research (NCTR) suggests that moderate to high doses of the drug may cause thyroid cancer in mice—a concern heightened by the fact that the U.S. Department of Agriculture found illegally high residues of sulfamethazine in some pork products," the notice said.

The majority of hogs on the U.S. market receive sulfa. Sulfamethazine, the leading sulfa drug, has been used for thirty years to treat respiratory diseases and promote faster weight gain in food animals. Animals are supposed to be taken off the drug fifteen days before slaughter to ensure that the meat contains no illegal residues.

"This may not get rid of all traces, however, if the animals have continued exposure in the environment (for example, in their feed troughs) or in their feed," the report said.

The FDA sent a letter on March 10, 1988, to sulfamethazine manufacturers to explain the situation and inform them that the agency would review all safety information on sulfamethazine while NCTR's data underwent peer review.

FDA Commissioner Frank E. Young, M.D., Ph.D., said that after studying the information presented at the hearings, the FDA might take one of two steps: lower the legal limit for sulfamethazine residues in pork or decide that the drug's use in food-producing animals is an imminent health hazard.

A year later, in March 1989, there was another report in *FDA Consumer,* under the byline of Frank E. Young:

Last year I discussed in this column FDA's role as an educator, helping to solve public health problems by providing information and guidance to consumers, health professionals, and FDA-regulated industry. This role is especially important when a problem is due to the way a health Product—a drug or medical device, for example—is used, and not to a flaw in the Product itself. Education often proves more effective in solving such problems than does regulatory or legal action.

I am pleased to be able to cite a recent success story in which FDA played a vital educational role. The story begins in March of last year, when FDA conducted a survey of milk from stores in 10 major cities across the country. Laboratory analysis found small residues of the veterinary antimicrobial sulfamethazine in 36 of 49 samples tested.

These findings were particularly disturbing for a number of reasons. First, it is illegal to use sulfamethazine in milk producing cows. So, even though 25 of the 36 positive samples were below 5 parts per billion (ppb)—amounts so small that the reliability of the results couldn't be guaranteed—the fact that any residues were showing up in milk was a sign of trouble.

Second, some people are allergic to sulfa drugs, including sulfamethazine.

Third, the safety of sulfamethazine for use in any food-producing animals had recently been called into question by a study just completed at FDA's National Center for Toxicological Research. The study found that sulfamethazine—used legally since the 1950s to treat respiratory and other diseases and promote faster weight gain in hogs, cattle, and other animals—produced cancerous tumors in mice and rats. The findings raised the question of whether the drug might cause cancer in humans as well. (That study is currently under review; if its findings are supported, FDA may need to modify or ban the use of sulfa drugs in food-producing animals.) It was particularly distressing that residues of the drug were turning up in such a basic food as milk consumed by almost all our children and most adults every day.

Based on the results of its survey, and on similar reports of sulfa residues in milk published in scientific and dairy industry journals, FDA considered its options. The problem was not use of an illegal drug but illegal use of a legal drug; in other words, a user problem. The solution, FDA believed, could best be found through educating dairy farmers and veterinarians. And that could best be done with the help of other organizations in both government and industry.

So, in early April FDA met with representatives of dairy trade associations, the American Veterinary Medical Association, and the National Conference on Interstate Milk Shipments (NCIMS), which represents the milk inspection agencies in all 50 states. As a result of the meeting, NCIMS established a task group to immediately develop and distribute to dairy farmers, veterinarians, and its own member agencies information about the sulfa residue problem. The information materials warned that use of sulfamethazine in milk cows was illegal, that milk containing even low levels of the drug would be rejected, that continued reports of residues could erode consumer confidence in the milk supply, and that those using the drug illegally could face fines and imprisonment.

FDA's Center for Veterinary Medicine and Center for Food Safety and Applied Nutrition also helped spread the word to state agencies, dairy industry groups, and veterinary associations, who, in turn, alerted their members.

Of course, while these educational efforts were going on, FDA and state milk officials were taking necessary regulatory steps as well. Milk testing was increased as FDA made a new, more sensitive test method available to state agencies and the dairy industry.

In July, FDA and the U.S. Department of Agriculture met with representatives of other government agencies and 20 drug industry organizations to discuss better ways to provide guidance to dairy farmers and veterinarians on proper drug usage. Meanwhile, milk testing continued, throughout the summer and into the fall.

In November, NCIMS asked the state milk inspection agencies to report the results of their testing to FDA. The findings from the 34 states that responded showed dramatic improvement in the residue situation. Of 2,207 raw milk samples tested from May through September, only 1.5 percent had sulfamethazine levels of 10 parts per billion or more, compared to 10 percent found by FDA in March. It was apparent that the prompt actions taken by FDA, NCIMS, the dairy industry, and veterinarians had resulted in an impressive decrease in the level of the drug in the nation's milk supply.

The survey results showed that sulfamethazine levels had decreased steadily after the educational (and regulatory) efforts began. The number of samples that tested positive (in any amount) decreased from 7 percent in May to 3 percent in September. The number with sulfamethazine above 10 ppb dropped from 3 percent in May to 1 percent in September. Naturally, milk found to contain any sulfamethazine residues was discarded to keep it from getting to stores.

The residue awareness program clearly shows how successfully government agencies, health professionals, and regulated industry can work together. By means of a cost-effective cooperative information program—coupled with a vigorous state enforcement effort—a potentially serious public health hazard was eliminated in a little over half a year. That's a case study in consumer protection from which we can all draw a lesson.[17]

The lesson I drew was that while Dr. Young, his colleagues, and the dairy industry were well intentioned and did take effective action, we have all been unknowingly exposed to sulfamethazine, an allergen and a cancer-causing agent, since 1950. In November 1989, after new animals tests showed that sulfamethazine caused cancerous tumors of the thyroid glands of rats and mice, Dr. Gerald B. Guest, director of the Center for Veterinary Medicine at the FDA, said: "We have several steps to complete, but I expect that in six months we will propose to withdraw this drug from the market."[18]

Two separate surveys of milk were done in December 1989, one by *The Wall Street Journal* and the Center for Science in the Public Interest, a Washington, D.C.-based consumer group. In the *Journal*'s test, which involved fifty retail samples collected in ten major cities, 38 percent were found to be contaminated with sulfamethazine, other sulfa drugs, or antibiotics. Of twenty off-the-shelf samples purchased by the consumer group in metropolitan Washington, 20 percent were found to be tainted with sulfa drugs, including sulfamethazine.[19] Still a third milk survey was done by WCBS-TV in New York at the beginning of 1990, with similar findings.[20]

The FDA, pressured by *The Wall Street Journal*'s findings, tested retail milk supplies in thirteen cities. The FDA survey initially found residues of animal drugs in 51 percent of the samples, using a rough testing procedure. The FDA later reported more sophisticated tests found all the milk samples to be residue free.[21]

HIDDEN HORMONES

The European Economic Community (EEC) began 1989 by banning $130 million worth of American beef imports. The reason: hormone implants. The Europeans vehemently object to the practice of implanting growth-hormone pellets in cattle.

The Americans claim that the EEC's refusal to purchase American meats treated with anabolic steroids was actually aimed at lowering surplus beef built up because of the European Economic Community's agricultural policies.

Europe's concern about implants surfaced after a scandal in Italy in which a baby-food manufacturer illegally injected hormones directly into the muscles of cattle. The baby food produced from this meat contained a concentrated dose of the drugs; infants of both sexes developed breasts, and some of the females began to menstruate.

It was the same drug—diethylstilbestrol, a female hormone—that was injected under the skin of cattle, chickens, and turkeys in the United States from 1947 to 1959 but was banned because it was found that humans were getting residues of the hormone in their poultry. It was still given to cattle in feed and, in pellet form, in their ears until 1970, when it was finally prohibited because it was known to be a carcinogen. As late as 1983, it was still being purchased on the black market, but the legal use has been stopped.

In the United States, the government permits cattle growers to use three hormones—testosterone, estradiol, and progesterone—and two synthetic hormones—zeranol and trenbolone acetate. Each makes cattle grow faster and bigger. The hormones are implanted under the skin of the animal's ear to provide a steady, small amount of the hormone. Very little of the drug remains in the meat, according to the FDA.[22] The hormones make a head of cattle two hundred to three hundred pounds heavier at slaughter, but still lean.

According to Dr. Gary C. Smith, head of the department of animal science at Texas A&M University, on the average, a three-ounce portion of beef that has been grown without added hormones will have 1.2 nanograms of estrogen. The same portion of beef grown with hormones will have 1.9 nanograms.

In 1989, controversy emerged over yet another hormone, bovine somatotropin (BGH), a genetically engineered growth hormone. The FDA has not allowed somatotropin to be used commercially but had been permitting the sale of milk from BGH-treated herds.[23] Experiments have shown that BGH increases milk production by 11 percent.[24]

Opponents of BGH, in a petition to the FDA, cited scientific evidence that the hormone reduces fertility of cows and increases their susceptibility to infections. They also said that several questions about the effects on human health have yet to be answered.[25] A veterinarian dismissed from the FDA, Richard J. Burroughs, said in an interview with the *New York Times* that because of the agency's eagerness to approve the drug, important flaws in safety studies submitted by manufacturers were dismissed by his superiors and potential hazards to people and cattle were not thoroughly assessed.

Two of the drug's four manufacturers, the Monsanto Company and the American Cyanamid Company, were quoted in the *Times* article pointing out that the federal review of bovine somatotropin, which began in 1985, had been "more thorough and critical than any ever conducted for an animal drug."[26]

Consumer groups, environmentalists, and small farmers may put a damper on what is predicted to be a $400 million somatotropin market in the mid-1990s.[27] The FDA maintains that BGH is safe in milk because it has always been present in milk. It is produced naturally by the cow's pituitary gland.

Five big supermarket companies have refused to carry milk from cows treated with the genetically engineered drug because of consumer concern about BGH's safety.[28]

ANIMAL DRUG RESIDUES AND CONTAMINANTS IN HUMAN FOOD

In January 1986, a House Government Operations subcommittee issued a report, based on an earlier hearing, on the safety of animal-drug residues in human food. In the report, the subcommittee accused the Food and Drug Administration of failing to protect consumers from traces of veterinary drugs that can turn up in meat, dairy products, and eggs. According to the subcommittee, the FDA is neglecting its legal obligations by allowing the sale of thousands of unapproved animal drugs. FDA officials and other authorities argue that it is impossible to monitor all of the drugs being used and that many are actually different versions of a drug.

The report said that highly toxic veterinary prescription drugs were being widely and illegally sold over the counter in blatant disregard of any public health consequences resulting from their misuse.

The committee recommended that the FDA reestablish an independent office authorized to ensure that all regulatory decisions regarding animal drugs sufficiently protect the consumers of animal-derived foods.

The committee said that the agency had failed to restrict or ban some drugs identified as causing tumors in animals and that the FDA should require companies to devise better methods of detecting residues of drugs in meat. In some cases, no methods of monitoring the retention of drugs in animal tissues have been developed.

"It is rather remarkable," said the report, "that biologically potent chemicals which are obtainable for medicinal reasons only on prescription by a licensed physician can be used freely in large quantities by persons without any proper training concerning the potential health hazards associated with the handling and consumption of large quantities of these hormonal substances. Such practices are difficult to control adequately on a nationwide basis in foodstuffs handled in interstate and intrastate commerce by thousands of individual producers in quantities of several million animals. . . ."

"*If a drug is found to cause cancer, is it supposed to be automatically banned from use in food-producing animals?*" (emphasis added) Dr. Gerald Guest, director of the FDA's Center for Veterinary Medicine was asked.[29]

"No, not necessarily," Dr. Guest answered. "A provision of the Delaney anti-cancer clause of the Food, Drug, and Cosmetic Act stipulates that a carcinogenic compound can be used in food-producing animals if the drug will not harm the animals and if 'no residue' of the compound will be found in any edible tissues of the animal when tested by the approved methods.

"But as analytical methods have become more sensitive over the years, the exception has become unworkable. Levels of residues that were so low they were previously undetectable can now be detected. So we have developed procedures and criteria to permit these exceedingly low levels of residues that present an insignificant risk of cancer to the public."

What does Dr. Guest believe is an insignificant-risk level?

"One in a million. This doesn't mean that one in every million people will contract cancer as a result of this regulation. Rather it represents a one in a million increase in risk over the normal risk of cancer over a life time. This is considered an insignificant level of risk."[30]

Again I ask: How much of a cancer-causing agent causes cancer?

Dr. Guest agrees that illegal use of veterinary drugs can be "an even greater threat to the public health than the illegal use of human drugs. What puts a different light on this issue is that use of illegal human drugs generally involves the consent of the persons involved. But the consumer of meat, milk, and eggs, has no way of knowing if hazardous substances are present in these foods, and no way of knowing if unapproved drugs have been used on the animals."[31]

What happens if a farmer is caught using illegal veterinary drugs?

If unsafe drug residues are found in a carcass, the carcass is removed from the slaughterhouse, and the USDA will sample the next five animals from that farm. Second, the FDA will send a regulatory letter to the farmer, outlining the violation and warning of more stringent legal action if steps are not taken to correct the problem.[32]

Ironically, the USDA now recognizes what a number of "organic" farmers have known—tender, healthy meat can be obtained from animals that eat a normal diet without growth hormones or antibiotics. The USDA released a five-year study by department researchers that reported low-fat, tender meat can be produced economically by raising ram lambs on a high-forage alfalfa diet. The scientists also said that production of young lean lamb might strengthen markets for domestic lamb. This would give a competitive edge, they said, over imported lamb.

PBBS IN ANIMAL FEED

While veterinary drugs are used deliberately, unintentional additives are also a problem and require vigilance on the part of regulators.

More than five years after what has been called the most costly and disastrous accidental contamination ever to occur in United States agriculture, measurable amounts of the toxic chemical known as PBB (polybrominated biphenyl) were detected in hundreds of tissue samples taken from adults across Michigan. The environmental contamination occurred in the summer of 1973, when an estimated thousand pounds of PBB in the form of a flame-retardant chemical, which was supposed to be used for fireproofing a variety of plastics, were inadvertently substituted for a chemical additive to be used in livestock feed.

The contaminated feed found its way to hundreds of farms and subsequently into millions of animals and finally into humans. One indication that something was wrong came from dairy farmers who noticed a marked decrease in milk production from their cows, the development of abnormal growths on hooves, and an increase in the number of aborted calves.

Unfortunately, it took seven months to find out what was happening, and during that period contaminated meat and dairy products had been marketed, mostly in Michigan. When the source of the problem finally was traced to PBB-contaminated feed, efforts were made to contain the spread of the toxic chemical, which can accumulate in animal fat, by the state-supervised destruction of more than 30,000 cattle, 1,470 sheep, 5,900 swine, and 1.5 million chickens.

In the late 1970s, reports in the scientific literature began surfacing regarding nervous-system aberrations, alterations in the functioning of the liver, and impaired immune defenses among farm residents who had been widely exposed to PBB in contaminated milk, meat, butter, eggs, and cheese from their own farms.

At around the same time, PBB was reported to have been discovered in serum specimens and in breast milk of urban Michigan residents. The finding of PBB in the body fluids of people far from areas where many farm products had been most heavily contaminated suggested that exposure to the chemical contaminant had occurred throughout the state.

Findings that PBBs were still in the bodies of Michigan people five years later, even in those who lived far from the farming areas, prompted a study by Mary S. Wolff, Ph.D., and her colleagues at the Environmental Sciences Laboratory of New York City's Mount Sinai School of Medicine. They found that contamination with PBB spared no section of Michigan, reaching into residents of urban areas and those living in the remote upper peninsula, as well as into farmers in the most heavily contaminated rural counties.

Calculations based on a representative cross-section of the population of Michigan indicated that approximately 97 percent of that state's residents had measurable PBB in their bodies.

Studies have shown that once PBB gets into human fat, its level does not decline significantly for at least six or seven years and probably much longer. The danger, if any, from persistent PBB levels in fat where it is stored and possibly in other tissues is not known.

But as Dean W. Roberts, M.D., of Hahnemann Medical College in Philadelphia indicated in an editorial in the *Journal of the American Medical Association* about the PBB disaster, the potential delayed effects from the storage of PBB in the human body are a matter of concern, particularly in light of recent findings showing that PBBs are capable of inducing liver tumors in laboratory rats.

Said Dr. Roberts: "In view of the carcinogenesis lag time of up to two or three decades, it will be important to monitor a sample of the exposed population over a prolonged period."

Dr. Roberts characterized the finding as dramatic and a reminder of "our vulnerability to the increasing number and volume of potentially toxic chemicals used in manufacturing, agriculture, pest control and food processing."

In an incident in 1989, thirty-two cows died in late April in Texas. Soon after, ten cows died in Louisiana. The dairy farmers involved sought help from government agents. State and federal inspectors found that a railroad car previously used to transport barium carbonate, a rat poison, had not been properly cleaned before animal feed was transported. Only milk from two herds was found to contain high levels of barium carbonate, and it was dumped.[33]

In still another incident in April 1989, inspectors from the United States Department of Agriculture discovered that samples of pork and sausage in Arkansas were contaminated with heptachlor, the cancer-causing pesticide banned eleven years before.[34] (See page 19 for more about heptachlor.)

In the case of the PPB disaster and the poisoned cows, it was the general public, not government inspectors, who first discovered the contamination. Since this is often the case, it is important that you, the consumer, be educated about food safety.

The first Meat Inspection Act, March 18, 1907, was put into force after the author Upton Sinclair revealed conditions in meat plants in his book *The Jungle*.

The meat bill passed on November 21, 1967, provided matching funds for states to improve their meat-inspection programs. It also:

- Extended the federal program to include commerce wholly within the District of Columbia or within any territory not having a legislative body.
- Prohibited commerce in animal products not intended for human use unless properly marked as inedible.
- Provided for record-keeping by certain slaughterers and handlers; registration and regulation of certain handlers of dead, dying, disabled, or diseased animals.
- Authorized regulation of meat storage and handling to prevent adulteration or misbranding.
- Provided for withdrawal or refusal of inspection service, for detention, seizure and condemnation, injunction and investigation as new enforcement tools.
- Subjected meat imports to the same requirements as those for domestic meats.

In a letter to the author, Senator Mondale said: "I am totally satisfied with the new [meat] law, and I feel that it was the best possible bill that could have been passed."[35]

But, unfortunately, there is still plenty of opportunity to slip adulterated meat onto the consumer's plate.

MEAT INSPECTION

The fact remains that federal inspection is no guarantee of clean meat today. Once a plant is in operation, every live animal is supposedly examined in its holding pen by a veterinarian or by an inspector supervised by a veterinarian. After slaughter, federal meat inspectors are supposed to examine each carcass, including internal organs and glands, to be sure that no unwholesome condition exists. A carcass that passes this inspection is stamped with a purple USDA shield mark.

During the production of processed meat, inspectors are supposed to examine both meat and nonmeat ingredients, and check a dozen or more steps to ensure that meat is wholesome and prepared according to approved formulas. They inspect curing solutions, check processing times and temperatures, and control the use of restricted ingredients. They must see that all containers are properly filled and labeled.

Sounds good on paper, doesn't it?

The U.S. inspection system depends on sight, smell, and touch, but none of these methods detects chemical residues such as antibiotics, bacteria, and microbiological toxins.

Laboratory tests are performed on only a tiny percentage of all animals.

The Federal Meat and Poultry Inspection program (of the FSIS) employs around seven thousand inspectors, down from ten thousand in 1980, to examine the carcasses of nearly 120 million cows, pigs, and horses and 5.6 billion chickens. Another twenty-one hundred inspectors are employed in state inspection programs.[36] The inspectors in the field check production at 6,578 slaughterhouses and processing plants.

Bruce Ingersoll, writing in the *Wall Street Journal,* May 16, 1989, offered a graphic description of what it is like to inspect meat:

> Down the slaughterhouse line they come, five heifer carcasses a minute, hour after hour. And under new procedures being tested here, a federal meat inspector has all of 12 seconds in which to examine each beast, inside and out, as it passes by.
>
> Not to worry: The U.S. Department of Agriculture has installed a long mirror so its inspectors, while they are at it, can glance at the backsides of the dead cattle for abscesses, grubs, and other parasites.
>
> But the looking glass is only a theoretical boon to beef inspection. "Have you ever tried to see anything in a mirror 15 feet away through steam and fog?" asks inspector Michael Anderson. "You just hope that what you may have missed wasn't major."

Out of his other eye, the inspector peers for a split-second into the abdominal cavity of each passing animal, checking the kidneys, particularly for signs of disease before the beef is ultimately given that reassuring USDA inspection stamp. Often, Mr. Anderson says, it is too dark in there "to see much of anything."

The USDA said that these new inspection procedures, proposed to save time and money, were as good as the old way, which was to split carcasses into sides of beef and twirl them around for easy close-up inspection. There was such an outcry after Ingersoll's article and other publicity about the USDA's new methods of inspection that it had to back down. The Agriculture Department, yielding to an uproar of consumer protests, withdrew its plans to reduce the frequency of meat and poultry inspections at most processing plants and to cut its force of food-safety inspectors.[37]

The USDA in 1988 proposed something that everyone liked: a requirement to identify all swine in interstate commerce in order to make it easier to trace the source of diseased animals or those with drug or chemical residues.[38] Assistant Secretary of Agriculture for Marketing and Inspection Services Kenneth A. Gilles said: "A nationwide identification and traceback system would provide the mechanism for tracing the source of contaminated food as well as the information necessary for pinpointing and correcting animal health problems. It also would benefit pork production by enhancing disease control to reduce losses."

Under the rule, the USDA expanded its requirements so that anyone handling swine in interstate commerce—from the farm to the meat plant—has to identify the animals and maintain records on that identification for two years.

"Such a system facilitates efforts to eradicate diseases by making it possible to trace movements of infected swine and thus locate sources of infection," Gilles said. "Without a comprehensive system, investigations are time-consuming and costly to state and federal agencies. The requirements increase efficiency and protect the public health."

More than seventy-seven million hogs a year are slaughtered under federal inspection.

CHICKEN INSPECTION

Americans consume more than four billion chickens every year.

In July 1989, a coalition of farmers, workers, and consumer groups issued a broad attack on chicken producers, saying that excessive speed on processing lines encourages bacteria contamination and aggravates health hazards for workers and consumers.[39]

"Americans eat more poultry than beef, and the poultry business rivals the old meatpackers as an industry out of control," said Meredith Emmett, executive director of the Institute for Southern Studies, a research group in Durham, North Carolina, that assembled the coalition.

Most of the accusations against the sixteen-billion-dollar industry were not new. But it was the first time the chicken industry received so much criticism from so many at one time. The critics attacked the growing concentration of the industry in the hands of a few major corporations. In 1960, 286 companies sold chickens commercially. Today there are only 47, and the market is dominated by a few giants including Tyson Foods, Conagra, Gold Kist, Holly Farms, and Perdue Farms. These companies receive many of their chickens from small farmers under contract to raise them.

Modern production lines for gutting chickens now move at a rate of seventy to ninety birds a minute, increasing the workers' repetitive movements. *Salmonella* is in about 37 percent of chickens approved by the USDA. That percentage increases with the speed of the production lines at slaughter plants, according to former USDA microbiologist Gerald Kuester.

Federal law mandates that inspectors observe every bird to detect lesions, bruises, or other signs of disease. An inspector has between one and three seconds to examine a bird, depending on the speed of the processing line, the committee reported. However, microbial organisms and chemical residues that may cause illness in humans cannot be detected in this manner.

Kuester accused the department of suppressing information that casts doubt on poultry's wholesomeness. He cited an unpublished 1987 study of a plant in Puerto Rico showing that 76 percent of the birds leaving the plant were tainted with *Salmonella*.

Salmonella and similar organisms are commonly found in fecal matter and frequently come in contact with the skin and flesh of chickens during operations to remove organs and feathers. Many carcasses are heavily contaminated with fecal flora, even when the carcasses appear clean to the naked eye.

Kuester particularly criticized the widespread industry practice of mingling tainted birds with clean ones in processing vats. "It's no different than sticking that bird in your toilet before you eat it," he said.[40]

The FSIS now analyzes chemical residues in a random sample of chickens, but the committee contended that the sample is too small to offer sufficient protection.

Government inspectors did not identify the chickens contaminated with heptachlor mentioned in chapter 2.

IMPROVING INSPECTION

Two years before the coalition issued its broadside against poultry inspection, the National Research Council, the principal operating agency of the National Academy of Sciences, reported on an eighteen-month study of meat and poultry inspection done at the request of the USDA.[41]

Current poultry inspection procedures, which emphasize bird-by-bird visual and manual examination, cannot detect the most important types of microbial or chemical contamination and therefore "cannot provide effective protection" for public health, the National Research Council concluded.

The NRC committee stated that the disease microorganisms *Salmonella* and *Campylobacter* are both present on a significant number of chickens at the time of slaughter and retail sale. These bacteria can cause stomach ache, diarrhea, and other food-poisoning symptoms unless the chicken is handled properly and cooked thoroughly. Chickens are not the only sources of these microorganisms, the committee pointed out, but they contribute to the overall problem.[42]

The committee urged the FSIS to work with other agencies to monitor feed, water, and the production environment for pathogens and chemicals that might taint poultry during the breeding, hatching, and growing periods. It also urged the USDA agency to include better microbial and chemical analysis of a random sampling of chickens at poultry processing plants.

The NRC suggested that the FSIS require labels on retail poultry products to alert the public to possible health risks and describe proper cooking and handling procedures. Education programs for workers in the poultry industry and commerical food establishments could also help reduce risk to consumers, the committee said.

Committee members emphasized that the public should not interpret their findings as a condemnation of poultry, which occupies an important place in the American diet. "Poultry is nutritious and a desirable part of the diet. We don't want to discourage anyone from eating chicken," commented committee chairman Joseph Rodricks of Environ Corporation, Washington, D.C. The committee advised consumers to keep raw poultry products properly refrigerated, to make sure that raw poultry does not come into contact with other foods in order to prevent cross-contamination, and to cook poultry products thoroughly.

The NRC committee stated that the number of meat samples containing illegal levels of antibiotic residues was "very high inded" for the samples tested from 1979 to 1983.

According to the NRC report, the USDA runs laboratory tests on only 1 percent of all carcasses.

Although chemical residues in poultry are potentially hazardous, the committee found no evidence that they present significant risk. It emphasized that not much is known about some classes of residues or the extent of their occurrence in chickens.

The committee recommended that the FSIS shift its focus from the present bird-by-bird inspection procedure to one based on random sampling of birds. It suggested a three-tier scheme that would begin with close examination of individual birds, followed by laboratory work to detect microorganisms, and some simple chemical tests at the plant. A smaller sample of chickens would then be frozen and sent to a central laboratory for more detailed studies.

To provide greater protection to the public, the committee also recommended that the FSIS aim at preventing contamination of chicken "as early as possible in the production process." It noted that achieving this goal will require "a concerted effort among responsible authorities" such as the Environmental Protection Agency, the Food and Drug Administration, and state and local health departments, since the FSIS does not have jurisdiction beyond the slaughterhouse.

FURTHER RESEARCH

The committee called on the FSIS to gather more data about chemical contaminants in poultry and to support epidemiologic surveys that tie the actual amount and type of microbial contamination in chicken to specific incidence of infection. One way to achieve this latter recommendation, it said, would be to develop a network of sentinel county health departments equipped with adequate laboratory facilities and located in areas where a few identified poultry plants supply all the chickens for local markets. These kinds of data can assist the inspection service in evaluating the effectiveness of current and innovative procedures, the committee pointed out.

Serving with Rodricks on the committee were vice-chairman John C. Bailar III, Harvard School of Public Health and Office of Disease Prevention and Health Promotion, U.S. Department of Health and Human Services; Thomas Grumbly, Health Effects Institute, Cambridge, Massachusetts; Miley W. Merkhofer, Applied Decision Analysis Inc., Menlo Park, California; J. Glenn Morris, School of Medicine, University of Maryland, Baltimore; Morris Potter, division of bacterial diseases, Centers for Disease Control, U.S. Public Health Service, Atlanta; and Michael Pullen, College of Veterinary Medicine, University of Minnesota, St. Paul.

The causes of increasing incidence of foodborne disease are diverse. Contributing factors include: The greater concentration of animals in larger production units, which permits easier transmission of disease from one animal to the other; the considerable geographic movement of animals and birds, which can spread disease across the countryside; the use of improperly processed animal byproducts and wastes in animal feeds, which can introduce and perpetuate a disease cycle; the concentration of animal slaughter in fewer and larger plants, which increases the possibility for cross-contamination between carcasses. In addition, the organisms themselves have been evolving. They are adapting to modern food processing and are more able to survive. Also, they are developing resistance to human drug therapies.

The increase in eating away from home means more mass production of food and greater inherent possibilities of improper heating and refrigeration. A Centers for Disease Control study of factors contributing to the increase of outbreaks of meat- and poultry-borne disease in humans found that improper cooling of food occurred in about half the outbreaks. Cooking food far in advance of eating it contributed to one-third of the outbreaks. Inadequate cooking contributed to one-fourth, while inadequate reheating or improper hot storage each contributed to about one-fifth of the outbreaks. If the raw meat and poultry had not been contaminated, of course, this improper heating and cooking would not have led to foodborne disease.

There is a ray of hope that may control *Salmonella* in poultry and meats purchased at the supermarket. Richard Whiting of the USDA Microbiological Food Safety Laboratory in Philadelphia, Pennsylvania, is working with a bacteria in water and soil that is a predator of *Salmonella*. The bacteria, *Bdellovibrio,* is apparently harmless to humans. Whiting said that the hope is that *Bdellovibrio* can be added to packages and will kill any *Salmonella* present. Whiting said that *Bdellovibrio* is now undergoing tests, and it will be at least two or three years before its practicality and safety will be known.[43]

WHAT CAN YOU DO TO PROTECT YOURSELF FROM ADULTERATED MEAT AND POULTRY?

In answer to this question, most health officers to whom I spoke said, "Nothing." They explained that there is no way in today's marketplace for a consumer to be sure that the meat or poultry purchased is wholesome. Sight and smell are no longer to be trusted because the chemicals that are in use today can doctor decaying, diseased, or just plain stale food. All consumers can do, they say, is to rely on the federal, state, or local inspectors, and put their faith in the brand name of the product and the store selling it.

However, it is apparent to me, after engaging in research for this book, that there *are* things that consumers can and should do to protect their food:

1. Report any sanitary violation found in a store and any contamination of packaged food discovered at home.

2. Report any outbreak of suspected foodborne illness in the family. (While most boards of health and other protective agencies may be too understaffed to search out abuses effectively, they usually are only too happy to follow through on a suspected offense.)

3. Urge any group you belong to to find out how your state is implementing poultry and meat inspection—or find out for yourself. Some states are sure to claim insufficient funds or insufficient personnel and will lag behind on food-inspection improvements.

4. Don't purchase any meat in a supermarket if its container has been damaged in any way.

5. Don't buy an unrefrigerated canned ham. Canned hams must be refrigerated at all times, and many supermarkets ignore this cardinal rule.

6. Don't contaminate the meat at home yourself. Fresh meat should be unwrapped as soon as it comes from the market. Store fresh meat uncovered or loosely covered in the coldest part of the refrigerator. Cured meat should also be stored in the refrigerator. Canned hams should be kept under refrigeration. Frozen meat should be stored at a temperature of 0°F or lower. It may be placed in the refrigerator under ordinary refrigeration if it is to be used immediately after defrosting. Never refreeze meat.

7. Do not leave frozen fowl unrefrigerated to defrost. Keep it in the refrigerator even if it takes several days for it to thaw.

8. Don't place other food in a container that previously held raw meat, and do not set other foods on a counter on which raw meat,

fish, or poultry has been placed without first disinfecting the counter with soap and water.

9. Wash your hands after touching raw meat.

10. Practice good hygiene. Wash your hands after going to the bathroom, and don't handle meat when you are ill with a contagious ailment, especially an infected finger.

11. Never, never eat raw or undercooked meat. Steak tartar and pink hamburger are items of the past.

12. Don't look for bargains. If meat, fish, or poultry in any form is being sold far below the normal price, there's a reason, and it is usually not for the benefit of the consumer.

13. Microwave: Carefully observe the cookbook standing time. Where full cooking is vital to kill disease-causing agents in meat and poultry, let the food stand outside the oven—preferably covered with foil to retain heat—for the full number of minutes recommended to complete cooking.

14. Refrigerate hot dogs and lunch meats in their original vacuum-sealed package for two weeks. Once you open the package, you should rewrap it well and plan to use the rest in three to five days.

15. To reach the USDA's Meat and Poultry Hotline, call (202) 472-4485. You can ask questions about the proper handling of meat and poultry and how to tell if they're safe to eat.

16. Ham slices or whole hams bought in paper or plastic wrap should be stored in the coldest part of the refrigerator. Ham slices should be used in three to four days, a whole ham within a week. Even most canned hams should be refrigerated. Read the label for storage time.

17. Stuff poultry just before you're ready to cook it, and stuff it loosely. This gives heat from the oven a better chance to cook the stuffing all the way through.

18. Hamburger receives more handling than does many other kinds of beef and is thus exposed to many of the common food poisoners, including salmonella and staph. So hamburgers should be cooked thoroughly; so should meat loaf. You can store hamburger in the coldest part of the refrigerator for use in a day or

two; otherwise, freeze it. It will keep frozen at full quality for three to four months.

JACK SPRAT AND MEAT AND POULTRY CHOICES

As for reducing what many consider to be one of the most dangerous "poisons" in meat and poultry, fat, here are some hints:

The National Research Council of the National Academy of Sciences recommended in 1988 that the federal government revise current regulations that govern grading, labeling, and product standards to provide a greater incentive for production and marketing of leaner meat and dairy products.[44]

Current meat-grading policies "encourage overfattening of beef and lamb," the committee found, while available labeling and nutrition information fail to inform consumers adequately about lower-fat animal products already available in the marketplace.

The "real solution" to excessive dietary fat, saturated fatty acids, and cholesterol "lies in the production of leaner animals," it said.

The committee said that available data showed that an estimated 70 percent of the saturated fatty acids in the diet comes from animal sources. By commodity, this includes 30 percent from millk and milk products; 25 percent from red meat, poultry, and fish; 10 percent from fats of animal origin (such as tallow for cooking); and 5 percent from eggs.

To understand "extra lean" and other fat claims on meat and poultry, see chapter 12.

WHAT YOU CAN DO TO LOWER THE FAT CONTENT OF POULTRY AND MEAT

- Before cooking, inspect the chicken and pull out any visible globules of yellow fat.
- Remove the skin before or after cooking. Many cooks find that flavor suffers if the skin is taken off before the bird goes into the oven or pan. But you can minimize the flavor loss after removing the skin by browning the meat in a small splash of vegetable oil and then cooking it slowly in broth, wine, or water. Keep it covered the whole time, letting it steep in its own juices.

- Eat white meat in preference to dark. One hundred grams of a mixture of light and dark meat contain 190 calories, according to USDA nutritionist Margaret Hoke; 35 percent of its calories are derived from fat. But the same weight of light meat alone contains 173 calories, only 23 percent of them from fat.
- Consider other light foods like turkey and fish. A hundred grams of white turkey meat has 157 calories, only 18 percent of them derived from fat. And the same serving of flounder, a deepsea fish, has about half the calories of chicken—98—and 11 percent of the calories come from fat.

5 ～ A Fish Story

A twenty-four-year-old New Yorker got more than he bargained for when his girlfriend invited him to her home for dinner. The day after the meal, he was admitted to the hospital with a ten-hour history of pain in his lower right side. The pain had not moved, although it had gradually intensified. There was no history of nausea, vomiting, or lack of appetite. On the day of admission, the young fellow had had two loose stools. Other than that, he appeared to be in perfect health with a regular heartbeat and normal blood pressure and temperature.[1]

He was observed by his physicians for six hours, after which he was again examined; the pain was still severe in his lower right side. "Appendicitis," the doctors agreed, but found during surgery that his appendix was perfectly normal. Just as they were about to sew the patient back up, one of the physicians noticed a pinkish-red "sinuous worm," about 4.2 centimeters long, crawling from the young man's abdomen onto the surgical drapes.

The nematode that crawled out of the patient belonged to the order *Dioctophymatoidea*. The physicians believe the patient had swallowed the worm with the sashimi and sushi (raw fish) meal his girlfriend had made after purchasing the fish at a neighborhood store.

This is just one of a growing list of parasitic diseases acquired by humans after the ingestion of infected fish that is raw or insufficiently cooked. Worms and other parasites are linked to many marine fish taken regularly off both coasts of the United States, as well as off Japan and Europe, by commercial fishermen. Surveys have shown that fish, including cod, whiting, haddock, herring, and salmon, are frequently infected. The consumption of these fish raw or after insufficient cooking, smoking, salting, or marinating may lead to one of several ailments, depending on whether the infection is localized to the stomach or to the small intestine.

In acute stomach worm infection, severe upper abdominal pain, nausea, and vomiting occur one to twelve hours after the consumption of infected raw fish. When a worm lodges in the lower intestines, however, it may not cause symptoms until up to a week later.

Such infections can be avoided by heating fish to at least 60° C or 140° F for five minutes or by freezing the fish at −20° C or −4° F for sixty hours. But as Steven Ostroff, M.D., an epidemiologist from the Communicable Disease Centers, said in an interview with the author, neither he nor any of his colleagues will eat raw fish, including shellfish, after what they have seen recently in their work.[2]

"It's like Russian roulette," he said. "It may not mean more than a bellyache to a healthy young adult, but to an AIDS victim or to others with weakened immune systems, raw fish should not be eaten at all. It could be fatal."

As for well-cooked, well-handled fish, that is a different story. In our hurry-up lives, fish is quick to prepare. Nutrition experts have encouraged us to eat fish as a more healthful alternative to red meat, and until recently, the eating of seafood was up significantly.[3] However, publicity about water pollution, oil spills, and contaminated fish has tended to discourage consumption.[4]

How can you tell if the fish you are eating or the clams you are swallowing really came from safe waters?

In the first edition of *Poisons in Your Food,* I wrote: "With increasingly polluted water and wider distribution of fish, it is imperative that the American consumer be protected against disease-bearing or low-quality fish.

"Many communities discharge human excrement into convenient rivers, lakes, or estuaries. It was always assumed that the contaminating material was naturally purified by dilution, aeration, exposure to sunlight, and microbial action. However, a researcher from the Biological Sciences Laboratory at Fort Detrick, in Frederick, Maryland, Werner A. Janssen, and a researcher from Chesapeake Biological Laboratory of the Natural Resources Institute, University of Maryland, Caldwell D. Meyers, found this was not true. They found that live fish may become infected with dangerous germs from man, and thus constitute a public health problem."[5]

The pollution situation today is as bad or even worse than it was in 1969. Beaches in the United States are closed periodically because the bacteria count is too high for human bathing.

What about the fish humans eat that are swimming in those waters?

The ability of shellfish to act as human disease carriers has been well documented. Early in this century the consumption of shellfish harvested from polluted water was shown to be the cause of typhoid fever outbreaks, and in the past ten years outbreaks of infectious hepatitis in this country and abroad have been associated with the consumption of raw oysters and clams.

This epidemiological evidence has been supported by a number of laboratory studies that have shown that oysters and clams will not only take up a significant amount of virus or bacteria from contaminated water, but will also concentrate these organisms to a level up to sixty times that found in the surrounding water. Contamination that occurs naturally with certain types of viruses has been found in oysters taken from water that, frankly, has been polluted with human wastes. Paradoxically, shellfish grow best in areas most likely to be contaminated with human waste.[6]

Herbert L. DuPont, M.D., of the University of Texas Health Science Center, said that the standards for harvesting shellfish today are established by state rules and regulation.

Numerous problems contribute to shellfish contamination. The existing policies are often neither followed nor adequately enforced. During peak demand shellfish are harvested from areas that are not approved (a practice known as "bootlegging") and less commonly, mollusks are temporarily maintained in contaminated water after harvesting (wet storage). Many shell-fish farmers furnish their products to a number of suppliers without adequate documentation of their origin, making later tracing impossible. Finally, the shellfish may not be properly handled or refrigerated after harvesting.

Policing fishermen from plying their trade in forbidden waters is not unlike trying to stop drug smugglers' boats from landing their illegal cargo. As a fisherwoman told me, "One tip-off is the black clothing bootleggers wear so that they can be more unobtrusive fishing at night in forbidden waters."[7]

An undercover investigation, "Operation Pearl," shows both the extent of bootlegging of fish from illegal waters and how difficult it is to stop.

Don Kraemer, the investigator for the FDA's New Orleans district office, who has been tracking the activities of Louisiana oyster dealers and fishermen for years, said that bootlegging has been rampant since 1985. Kraemer estimated that 20 percent of the shellfish leaving Louisiana are from polluted waters.

State authorities, with 3.5 million acres of shellfish-growing areas and only a small water-patrol force, have not been able to contain the problem. Initial attempts to gather enough evidence to serve federal warrants on the dealers were unsuccessful, and in 1986 Kraemer suggested that a full-scale undercover operation would be the only way to prove violations of the Lacey Act, a federal law that makes it illegal to sell or receive illegally harvested shellfish in interstate commerce.

Bags of oysters are supposed to be tagged with their area of origin so that they can be traced if there is any problem with them. An undercover FDA agent, posing as a fisherman, purchased a bag of oysters from a reputable dealer, removed the tag, and hauled the oysters to dealers suspected of trading in illegal shellfish.

"I almost got caught out there," he told the dealers, implying he had harvested the oysters from a closed bay.

"We can't put that area tag on the oysters," the dealer would usually respond, and tag it instead with another area.

With these transactions, the FDA was able to document that, in violation of state law, the dealers:

- Purchased sacks of untagged oysters.
- Purchased oysters understood to be from a closed area.
- Falsified information on the tags.

To document interstate violations, the FDA enlisted the aid of the National Marine Fisheries Service. FDA investigators targeted the black-market dealers who routinely sell seafood out of state. The government investigators placed orders with these dealers through the seafood companies that National Marine Fisheries Service formed for use in undercover operations. The dealers sold and shipped the oysters.

On September 1, 1988, a combined federal-state strike force served ten search warrants on oyster dealers in Louisiana and Florida and nine arrest warrants on clam dealers in South Carolina. One South Carolina dealer is alleged to have sold more than $1 million worth of illegally obtained clams in a year. The fishermen were shipping and selling their catch mainly in southern and eastern states.

One FDA official speculates that an outbreak of hepatitis may have been linked to illegally harvested Florida shellfish.

Now that the task force is gone, do you think the bootleggers are back? After they were caught, they were subjected to fines of up to $20,000 and up to five years in jail.

Since the patrol force is small and the potential punishment rather light, what's to stop the illegal harvesting of shellfish from resuming?

Kraemer believes dealers will be more cautious about buying contaminated shellfish; this, in turn, will discourage fishermen fond of fishing in closed waters. But bootlegging is rampant along coastal areas. On July 22, 1989, for example, four persons were arrested in New Jersey at 1:00 A.M. They were transferring thousands of clams from one unrefrigerated pickup truck to another. The clams, if they had not been seized, would have been distributed to restaurants in Pennsylvania.[8]

New York has its own problems with bootleggers (see the Norwalk virus incident below).

Fish is even more perishable than meat and poultry and requires special handling from the time it is caught until the time it reaches the consumer. A major reason is that fish are caught at sea and die as they are brought aboard. And from that moment on they must be handled carefully and preserved on ice or by freezing and brought ashore.

HOW CONTAMINANTS GET IN THE WATER

How do contaminants get into the nation's waterways and oceans? There are a variety of ways but they all can be put into one of three categories.

- Point sources—generally pipes, which most often lead from municipal and industrial waste treatment plants. Considerable progress has been made in recent years in controlling discharges of contaminants from these plants.
- Nonpoint sources—broad paths by which rainfall or melting snows can either flush contaminants into waterways or soak them through the soil into groundwater supplies, which then seep into surface waterways. Runoff from nonpoint sources such as farms, feed lots, and city streets is an increasing source of aquatic contaminants. Other nonpoint sources include forest and mining operations and landfills.
- Atmospheric deposition (through the air)—acid rain, dust particles, and snowfall can deliver toxins to the water and consequently the fish. Although scientists know less about atmospheric deposits than about other contaminant sources, it seems to explain why high levels of certain contaminants are found in remote areas long distances from other possible sources.

Depending on where they live, fin fish and shellfish may be subjected to a variety of contaminants in their watery environment. Molly Joel Coye, M.D., Master of Public Health (M.P.H.), New Jersey state commissioner of health, and Marcia Goldoft, M.D., M.P.H., a research scientist in the state's health department, writing in *New Jersey Medicine* in July 1989, pointed out: "The high number of necessary tests to cover possible pathogens and the lack of tests for certain pathogens, such as Norwalk-type agents, make environmental sampling for pathogens a formidable task. Assessing water quality, therefore, depends on measuring indicator organisms rather than actual pathogens. The most commonly used indicator organisms are coliform bacteria, present in the intestines of warm-blooded animals."

They said that at present, all New Jersey sewage treatment plants with ocean outfall pipes discharge chlorinated effluents. These effluents contain intestinal microorganisms resistant to chlorine, primarily viruses. If ingestion of sewage-contaminated water should take place, the most typical health outcome would be acute stomach upset with nausea, vomiting, diarrhea, and fever occurring within several days of exposure. The same syndrome results when the causative organisms are transmitted by contaminated food.

The study of stomach viruses is in its infancy, according to Herbert L. DuPont, who says that state laboratories lack the ability to detect viruses in water, in shellfish, and in patients. In addition, he says, studies show that the absence of fecal coliform bacteria (the presence of which is a danger signal) in harvesting areas is an inadequate indicator of safety from virus contamination among shellfish.[9]

Late in 1987 the Environmental Protection Agency reported that one-quarter of United States lakes, rivers, and estuaries don't meet the objectives of the Clean Water Act. In many cases, coastal waters and inland lakes and rivers have been closed to both fishing and swimming. More important from the standpoint of the nation's seafood supply, the ability of fish stocks to reproduce continues to be jeopardized.

What can you catch from your "catch" of the day?

U.S. Centers for Disease Control in Atlanta reports that the most common illnesses linked to seafood are ciguatera and scombroid poisoning. Both toxins are found in the muscles of fish.

SCOMBROID POISONING

Between 1973 and 1986, 178 outbreaks of scombroid poisoning affecting 1,096 persons were reported to Centers for Disease Control. Outbreaks were reported from thirty states and the District of Columbia. Hawaii reported the largest number of outbreaks, 51, followed by California with 24. The most common reported fish were mahimahi (dolphin fish), tuna, and bluefish, but scombroid is also common in swordfish, mackerel, and bonito. Scombroid is in those fish only if they haven't been properly refrigerated and have been allowed to decompose. Illness begins minutes to hours after ingestion of the toxic fish. Symptoms resemble an allergic (histamine) reaction that frequently includes dizziness, headache, diarrhea, and a burning sensation or peppery taste in the mouth. Facial flushing, irregular heartbeat, itching, asthmalike symptoms, muscular weakness, and paralysis may also occur.[10]

The following are case histories of recent scombroid poisonings tracked down by state health departments:

On February 26, 1988, five patrons and three employees of a private club who had eaten a buffet lunch became ill. Six of the ill persons experienced symptoms that included headache, nausea, flushing, dizziness, and diarrhea ninety minutes after the meal. Investigation by the Illinois Department of Public Health revealed that seven of the ill persons had eaten mahimahi with dill sauce. The eighth had eaten the dill sauce scraped from the serving pan that held the fish.

The club had purchased 10.5 pounds of frozen mahimahi from a suburban Chicago distributor the week before it was served. The fish had been kept in the club's freezer until February 26, when it was thawed by placing under running water for fifteen minutes. The fish was then cut into portions, placed flat in pans in the cooler, and baked as needed during the lunch hour until the supply was depleted.

Seven months later, nine cases of scombroid fish poisoning in Charleston, West Virginia, were investigated. Of the nine, five occurred after consumption of a midday meal at a restaurant on September 9, one case followed an evening meal at a second restaurant, and three cases occurred after an evening meal of fish prepared at home but obtained from the first restaurant. The patients ranged in age from eighteen to sixty-four years. Symptoms began from five to sixty minutes after the meal. Five patients required emergency room treatment and one was admitted for observation because of a cardiac condition.

It was determined that the source of the outbreaks in Chicago and West Virginia was yellowfin tuna, probably caught one day before purchase in waters off the coast of New Jersey, Rhode Island, or

West Virginia. It had been packed in ice on the boat. The tuna was then placed on the docks in Cape May or Barnegat Light, again packed in ice, and delivered by truck to Philadelphia . . . where the fish was divided and repacked in ice for shipment to wholesalers. The tuna left the Philadelphia supply plant by refrigerated truck twelve hours after arrival. The wholesaler in Charleston received 188 pounds of yellowfin tuna by truck one day before the outbreak. The wholesaler processed the tuna into steaks and shipped seventeen pounds of steaks from the same fish to each of the two restaurants implicated in the outbreaks.

Somewhere along the line, the temperature control broke down; experimental studies have shown that at refrigerator and freezing temperatures, histamine formation causing scombroid poisoning is negligible. Fish have to be kept on ice from the time they are caught until they are cooked. As the outbreaks described above illustrate, *cooking* toxic fish is not protective.

Ciguatera

On the other hand, neither preservation nor preparation procedures can prevent another toxin, ciguatera, which affects reef-dwelling fish in subtropical and tropical climates. More than four hundred species have been implicated, but only a few, such as barracuda and red snapper, are of commercial significance, and the toxin only rarely affects the subtropical United States fish eater. The toxin becomes concentrated as it moves up the food chain, and people who have a preference for liver, brains, or eyes of fish are at the greatest risk. Ciguatera poisoning causes cramps, vomiting, diarrhea, and progressive numbness and burning sensations that generally begin in the mouth and throat. In severe cases, the central nervous system, heart, and respiratory system are affected. For months afterward, unusual sensory phenomena may keep a person from going to work.[11]

PARALYTIC SHELLFISH POISONING

Humans have been and can be poisoned from eating toxic shellfish in many places throughout the world.[12] Toxins that cause potentially fatal paralytic shellfish poisoning (PSP) are produced by microscopic algae called dinoflagellates. From June through October—especially on the Pacific and New England coasts—mussels, clams, oysters, and scallops may ingest poison-producing dinoflagellates, tiny organisms that produce "red tides" (although not all red tides are produced by poison-producing dinoflagellates). The nerve poison is resistant to cooking. The earliest symptoms, numbness around the mouth, appear five to thirty minutes after eating. Then nausea, vomiting, and abdominal cramps develop, followed by muscle weakness and paralysis. Respiratory failure may cause death.

An increasing number of paralytic shellfish poisoning episodes have occurred in New England coastal areas, and PSP seems to be spreading farther south into Long Island Sound and the Middle Atlantic states. John Pearce, deputy director, National Marine Fisheries, said in 1989 that the spread of the poisonous "cells" is associated with "some form of environmental change" in the coastal marine waters. Referring to the "red," "brown," and "green tides," Pearce said that such events have been particularly common in Raritan Bay, Long Island Sound, and Chesapeake Bay, but they are also being found offshore over the continental shelf during July and August.[13]

The colorful tides result from frequent plankton blooms (algae), which are fed by nutrients from sewage and sludge discharges in the ocean, as well as from nitrogen and phosphorous entering coastal waters.

VIBRIO VULNIFICUS

National Institutes of Health–supported research scientists began warning physicians in mid-Atlantic coastal areas that they should be aware of an unusually virulent marine bacterium, *Vibrio vulnificus*.[14] It causes problems mainly in undercooked shellfish.

James D. Oliver, Ph.D., and colleagues in the department of biology, University of North Carolina at Charlotte, working under a National Institutes of Health (NIH) grant, isolated 3,887 *Vibrios* from sea water, sediment, plankton, and animal samples taken from eighty sites ranging from Miami to Portland, Maine. In the study,

33 isolates were almost identical to clinical strains of *Vibrio vulnificus* studied by the Centers for Disease Control in Atlanta.

Although *V. vulnificus* occurs in relatively small numbers, it causes severe illness in humans and is fatal nearly 50 percent of the time. When ingested in fish or seawater, it can cause severe low blood pressure, shock, and blood poisoning. In 1987, three people died from oysters contaminated with *Vibrio vulnificus,* and each year the state of Florida reports five or six deaths from this bacteria in seafood.[15]

CHOLERA

Cholera is an acute infection involving the entire small bowel and is characterized by profuse watery diarrhea, vomiting, muscular cramps, dehydration, and collapse. The causative organism is *Vibrio cholerae,* and susceptibility to it varies among individuals since some people have a natural immunity. Cholera is spread by ingestion of water, seafoods, and other foods contaminated by the excrement of persons who have the infection. It is endemic in countries from which we import food, such as some in Asia and Africa, and also along the Gulf Coast of the United States.[16]

In 1986, twenty people were known to have contracted cholera and one person died from eating cholera-contaminated shellfish, according to the Communicable Disease Centers.

LISTERIA

Although tests for this bacteria on raw seafood had never been done, and no reports of problems with *Listeria*-contaminated shellfish had been made, FDA researchers had reason to suspect it might show up in raw fish.

As Steven Weagant of the FDA noted, *Listeria monocytogenes* thrives in the kind of cold, moist environment that processing conditions for raw fish and some other foods provide. Contaminated bacteria in soft cheese was responsible for the deaths of forty-seven people in southern California four years ago. Other outbreaks of listeriosis, the disease caused by *Listeria,* were associated with consuming contaminated coleslaw and pasteurized milk that became contaminated after pasteurization. (See pages 154 and 155.)

Symptoms of listeriosis include fever, headache, nausea, and vomiting. The infection is especially dangerous in the elderly, in people with weakened immune systems (such as AIDS patients and those on cancer chemotherapy) and in pregnant women (because of risk to the fetus). Weagant and his colleagues felt uneasy about the role of this potentially deadly bacteria in food and in June 1987 added a check for *Listeria* to the standard battery of tests run on shrimp imported from Taiwan.

Listeria monocytogenes was found in fifteen of fifty-seven samples. Two of the positive samples were raw shrimp. (No illnesses were reported from consumption of any seafood.)

The FDA did not remove the shrimp from the market because the FDA determined it was "OK as long as it was properly cooked." Susan McCarthy, a Fishery Research Branch microbiologist, designed an experiment to compare the boiling time required to kill *Listeria* in contaminated shrimp harvested from the water with the time required to kill the bacteria in shrimp that have been injected with *Listeria* in the laboratory.

The experiment involved boiling both batches of shrimp for various intervals of from one to five minutes. Then, to determine whether any *Listeria* damaged by the boiling could recover, she incubated cells from the shrimp at temperatures favorable to *Listeria* growth. Bacteria from the injected shrimp were able to recover even after being boiled for five minutes. However, after only one minute's boiling, none of the bacteria in the naturally contaminated shrimp survived.

The shorter time needed to kill the bacteria in the naturally contaminated shrimp suggested to FDA scientists that *Listeria* may be present only on the surface of the shellfish. Based on the laboratory findings, the researchers recommended that consumers eat only shrimp that has been boiled for at least one minute.[17]

Did you know that? Did those who ate *Listeria*-contaminated shrimp know that?

HEPATITIS

An inflammatory infection of the liver, hepatitis A virus spreads by fecal contamination and water; foodborne epidemics of hepatitis are common. Shellfish, particularly, is responsible. Hepatitis A has an incubation period of about two weeks and symptoms vary from a minor flulike illness to fatal liver failure, depending upon the victim's immunity. When you hear that there is a high coliform count in the ocean or lake in your area, it means that there is a high level of fecal contamination and, of course, an increased danger of hepatitis, among other ills.

NORWALK VIRUS

Norwalk virus causes about 40 percent of nonbacterial diarrhea in children and adults.[18] This is what we most often call "intestinal flu." Norwalk virus was documented in a major study conducted by Dr. Dale L. Mose, director of the Bureau of Communicable Disease Control of the New York State Department of Health in Albany, and ten of his colleagues. They collected data relating to 103 confirmed outbreaks of gastroenteritis in twenty-one countries, outbreaks that affected 1,017 persons from May through December 1982. The researchers reported that in contrast to previous sporadic outbreaks of gastroenteritis traced to raw shellfish consumption, the cases they investigated were frequent and widespread. While symptoms reportedly persisted less than forty-eight hours in most patients, 5 percent of those interviewed were ill for up to one week. The researchers were particularly surprised by the high attack rate—26 percent among persons who had eaten *steamed* clams—but not *raw* shellfish.

Tracing the source of shellfish implicated in the 1982 outbreaks, the investigators found that in addition to coming from New York waters, the shellfish came from Rhode Island, Massachusetts, North Carolina, and the Canadian province of Prince Edward Island.[19] From 1983 through 1985, 59 outbreaks involving 888 documented illnesses were investigated by New York State health officials. New Jersey had a large number of shellfish-related gastroenteritis outbreaks in 1983 and illnesses were documented in other states in the Northeast as well. Reports from Hawaii linked an illness to raw clams in 1983.

The incubation period for Norwalk virus is twenty-four to forty-eight hours. Symptoms include vomiting and diarrhea and last for twelve to sixty hours. Because the illness caused by Norwalk virus is usually mild and self-limiting, those affected may not even seek medical care. This makes areas contaminated with Norwalk virus difficult for public health officials to identify.

(There is, as of this writing, no way to test for Norwalk virus in water, but there are tests for human waste pollution that signifies unsafe waters.)

New York State health officials advised against eating raw shellfish. They said, in effect, that there are too many holes in the safety net. Clams and oysters from contaminated waters are reaching the public.

"We've had a number of outbreaks in different areas of the state where the clams or oysters were supposedly harvested legally and certified as 'OK,' " the health department officials noted. "It's been difficult at times to track the clams back to their origin and at times other clams or oysters have been mixed as the shellfish went through various stages of processing."

Viruses do get killed by proper cooking, but a number of tests have shown that "steamed clams" and sometimes shrimp are not cooked long enough.

BOTULINUS

A primary concern of the FDA is the discovery of *Clostridium botulinum* spores in fish packed under vacuum or in nitrogen or carbon dioxide to retard spoilage. Time and temperature abuse of these products can lead to the growth of the bacteria and toxin production.

So far, there are no reports of vacuum-packed fish causing botulism, but on November 2, 1987, the U.S. Centers for Disease

Control notified the FDA's Division of Emergency and Epidemiological Operations that a man and his nine-year-old son had been admitted to a hospital the previous evening with symptoms of botulism. Those symptoms included abdominal pain, vomiting, diarrhea, and blurred vision. They had reported eating a kapchunka, a whitefish prepared by a Russian method in which the uneviscerated fish is salted and then dried at room temperature. The kapchunka was purchased at a store in Forest Hills, New York.

The FDA's New York district office, in cooperation with New York City and state officials, immediately started an investigation, and by the next day, the fish suspected of causing the illnesses was identified as kapchunka. Working together, the officials got all the kapchunka off the market within two days.

On November 3, however, the FDA and the Communicable Disease Centers in Atlanta were notified of botulism poisoning in six people in Israel who had eaten a fish referred to as "rybetz," another name for kapchunka, as it was later learned. One of them, a seventy-seven-year-old woman, died thirty-six hours after eating the fish. Others who ate the fish became ill but recovered. Visitors to the United States from Israel had purchased the fish in Brooklyn and taken it back home in their flight carry-on luggage.

The Israeli Ministry of Health, the American embassy, and the FDA's International Affairs Staff worked to bring the tainted fish sample back to the United States for analysis. Both countries were extremely concerned about transporting the sample batch because it contained large amounts of the extremely deadly botulin toxin.

Unexpectedly, a second sample was also brought back—this by someone who turned two fish into authorities after hearing Israeli press reports about the botulism incident. Those fish, too, had been purchased in New York and transported to Israel.

By November 4, the FDA and the New York State Department of Agriculture and Markets had inspected Arthur's Smoked Fish, the firm that processed the fish, and Gold Star Smoked Fish, the distributor—both located in Brooklyn. During the inspections, the state agency seized all kapchunka at the firms, totaling about twenty-two hundred pounds.

The FDA's investigation was complicated by a language barrier and by various names that the fish was called. Because of the confusion, FDA inspectors visited all twenty-two stores that had received the uneviscerated fish from Gold Star Smoked Fish and collected fifty-one samples of several types of product.

Arthur's Smoked Fish's license had been revoked in June 1987, but was reinstated in August after the firm passed a New York State inspection.

All kapchunka was recalled from the market and the state called for new regulations to prohibit the sale, production, and distribution of all uneviscerated, salt-cured, air-dried fish, including kapchunka.

The FDA banned the interstate sale of kapchunka based on three deaths in New York State and the determination that kapchunka could not be processed safely.

CONTAMINATION

We don't only have to worry about bacteria and viruses in our water and fish; fish can be exposed to toxic chemicals such as mercury, lead, cadmium, polyether compounds, polychlorinated biphenyls (PCBs), and pesticides, including DDT.

On June 13, 1989, the Environmental Protection Agency reported that 17,365 different segments of surface water in forty-nine states and six territories were contaminated by toxic pollution, conventional pollution like sewage, or both.[20] These segments account for about 10 percent of the nation's river, stream, and coastal water mileage and lake and estuary area.

Of the polluted waters, 595 segments averaging six to ten miles each were contaminated by one or more of the 126 different toxic chemicals and metals from factories, sewage plants, and other specific sources. At a briefing, agency officials said that the toxic pollution threatened aquatic life and tended to build up in the food chain and concentrate in fish. They also said that the number of contaminated waterways was probably much higher because many of the chemicals not included on the list of 126 could poison surface water.

Of the polluters dumping toxic substances into the nation's waterways, 627 were industrial sources, including metal finishing and manufacturing plants, pulp and paper mills, petroleum refining plants, organic chemicals and plastics and synthetic plants; there were also twelve federal installations on the list of polluters, including military bases and Department of Energy nuclear plants, and 240 municipalities. The EPA's listed polluters are required to meet the water quality standards to be set by their states by June 4, 1992. If they do not, they will be subject to fines and other penalties.

Contamination of Lake Michigan

Lake Michigan is one of the prime examples of what our civilization has done to our waters, our fish, and ourselves.

The contamination of some Lake Michigan sport fish by toxic chemicals has been found to pose an increased risk of cancer among people who eat them, according to a report by the National Wildlife Federation. Researchers studied only Lake Michigan because it is the most heavily industrialized of the Great Lakes and because more data is available on it than on the other lakes.[21]

In the report, the National Wildlife Federation argues that the problem of toxic pollution in Lake Michigan fish is more serious than was previously reported.

The federation's report calculates the relative risk of cancer that accrues as a result of eating, over a lifetime, varying quantities of certain popular sport fish, including lake and brown trout, chinook and coho salmon, walleye and yellow perch. These fish have been found to be contaminated by four toxic chemicals persistent in Lake Michigan and the rest of the Great Lakes Basin. The fish are contaminated with chemicals such as polychlorinated biphenyls and the pesticides DDT, dieldrin, and chlordane. In laboratory experiments on animals, these substances have been associated with a range of adverse health effects, including cancer.

Among other things, the report suggests that the risk of cancer is significantly higher from consuming contaminated Great Lakes fish than it is from eating lobster or flounder from contaminated waters in Quincy Bay, Massachusetts, or salmon or Pacific cod from Puget Sound, Washington.

The federation calculates that a person who, over a lifetime, eats just seven meals of lake trout measuring between ten and twenty inches in length is running a 1-in-100,000 risk of getting cancer, a level of risk commonly used by government agencies in setting pollution controls. By these calculations the risk level increases along with the amount of fish consumed. A person who eats as many as seventy meals of Lake Michigan trout over his lifetime runs a much higher risk of 1 in 10,000, the federation concludes.

Officials say that most of the fish harvested commercially in Lake Michigan are whitefish that don't have significant levels of chemical contaminants.

In general, state advisories for Lake Michigan recommend that people not eat bottom feeders like carp and catfish, and larger fish of certain species such as lake trout, chinook, and brown trout. Beyond that, people are advised to reduce their consumption to no more than one meal of such fish per week.

The state warnings, like the Wildlife Federation's, urge that nursing mothers, pregnant women, women who expect to bear children, and children under the age of fifteen not eat any of the fish listed in the advisories.

Recent studies have detected an increase in birth defects among fish-eating birds. However, there is, as yet, little evidence of the effect such chemicals may have on humans eating contaminated fish.

Game Fish and Mercury

The FDA set limits for mercury in foods in 1969, after 120 people in Nigata, Japan, had fallen ill from eating fish contaminated with high amounts of mercury. Birth defects in offspring of some mothers in the group affected were also ascribed to mercury poisoning. Mercury, sometimes called "quicksilver," poisons the brain, liver, and kidney when absorbed in sufficient amounts. How much is enough to cause damage? This is still a matter of controversy.

The FDA instituted a nationwide testing program after it was discovered that tuna and swordfish on the American market had too much mercury. More than a million cans of tuna were recalled and, in 1971, the FDA forced the withdrawal of swordfish from commerce because of mercury contamination.[22]

Today, decades later, there is still a problem with mercury in fish. Between July 1 and December 31, 1986, the FDA checked 127 swordfish shipments from fifteen countries for mercury. Samples from over 70 percent had illegal levels. Currently, swordfish imports are automatically detained until they are shown to meet the FDA's requirements.[23]

What about domestic fish? Early in March 1989, the Florida Department of Health issued warnings against eating largemouth bass and warmouth caught in the western part of Palm Beach and in Broward and Dade counties.[24] Fish samples contained up to 4.4 ppm (parts per million) of methyl mercury, more than four times what the federal government considers safe. That's one of the highest concentrations ever recorded in the country.

Theories about how mercury got in the water range from wind-blown mercury-laden factory smoke to midnight dumpers.

Dioxin

Dioxin forms during the manufacture of chemicals such as those used in certain pesticides and during the chlorine bleaching process applied to paper, including paper products used with some foods, such as coffee filters and paper plates (see page 61).

Dioxin, even in small doses, causes cancer in animals. A major food source of dioxin for Americans is bottom fish from the Great Lakes, an area of the country with a great deal of industrial activity and chemical production.[25]

Two federal studies have confirmed fears that many paper mills are discharging dioxin into rivers and that the toxic chemical is accumulating in fish downstream. One of the studies by the EPA found that fish downstream from twenty-one of the eighty-one mills that were examined contained levels of dioxin far exceeding those the federal authorities have designated as hazardous.

A second EPA study found that the amount of dioxin in waste water in fifty-nine of the seventy-four mills examined was, although minute, far above the EPA standard for clean water.

Are there paper mills in your area? Who is checking the water and the fish?

Polychlorinated Biphenyls (PCBs)

PCBs were widely used until 1977 as electrical insulators in power transformers and other electrical devices. PCBs are no longer produced because they were found to cause liver tumors and reproductive problems in animals but they "live on" in our waters and in our food chain.

According to the FDA publication *FDA Consumer,* "Because PCBs persist in soild and sediment in water, occasional contamination of food may be unavoidable. Further, they can't be eliminated from food by processing. To limit consumers' exposure, FDA has established tolerances for PCBs in susceptible foods and in paper food-packaging material. The most significant food source for PCB residues is fish, primarily freshwater fish such as coho and chinook salmon from the Great Lakes, and bottom-feeding freshwater species from waters near other industrial areas—although coastal marine species may also contain PCBs. The State of New York closed some highly contaminated areas of the Hudson River to commercial fishing of striped bass because of PCBs."[26]

In 1989, New York fishermen instituted a suit against General Electric Company for damages stemming from toxic chemical contamination of the Hudson River. Fishermen can no longer fish for striped bass and trout for commercial or recreational purposes because of PCB contamination. The company stopped dumping PCBs into the river in 1977 after New York State's Department of Environmental Conservation found GE responsible for the presence of toxic chemicals.[27]

FISH FARMING

Since the first edition of *Poisons in Your Food* appeared, a new industry—fish farming—has emerged because of the dangers of pollution in lakes, streams, and oceans and because of competition for scarce fish. Aquatic farms produced 790 million pounds of fish and other seafood in 1988, or nearly 10 percent of the 8.1 billion pounds of fish and seafood consumed in the United States, the United States Department of Agriculture says.[28]

The consumption of catfish is rapidly increasing in popularity in this country, exceeding two hundred million pounds a year. Raised in hundreds of thousands of acres of farm ponds in the southern United States, these catfish are a white-fleshed fish with a mild flavor, rather than the taste of the muddy river bottom that the wild variety has.

In addition to most of our catfish and crayfish, American aquaculture is producing nearly all of our rainbow trout and 40 percent of our oysters. In other countries as well, aquaculture is giving a boost to fish and seafood supplies. Salmon is being farmed in Norway, Chile, New Zealand, and British Columbia, as well as in our own Pacific Northwest. Shrimp are being raised by farm production in areas as diverse as Ecuador and Southeast Asia.

Fish farming is not without its critics. Clashes have arisen over salmon farming in Puget Sound as well as trout farming and catfish farming because of the use of synthetic substances to control disease. Fungus, aquatic weeds, and other threats to farm-raised fish thrive more readily in fresh water than in saltwater. Some scientists are saying that antibiotics used in salmon farming and other fish farming can be absorbed into shellfish and other organisms and make some bacteria resistant to the drugs. Three antibiotics are now approved by the FDA for use on fish farms. The most commonly used is oxytetracycline (see page 95). Fish farmers are required to stop using medicated feed weeks before salmon are sent to market so that residues will not be present in the meat.

Studies have shown, however, that 90 percent of the antibiotics fed to fish are excreted in the feces. Last year researchers in Norway, the world's largest producer of farmed salmon, found that oxytetracycline persisted for months in the sediments below fish farms. Other studies have determined that aquatic bacteria develop resistance to the drugs. Of particular concern to health specialists is the possibility that resistances to antibiotics can be transferred from bacteria that cause fish diseases to bacteria that cause illnesses in people (see pages 94–97).

The FDA has already brought its first case against a Washington State company for selling unapproved drugs for use in raising food fish.[29] But your chances of getting wholesome, nutritious fish from a carefully run farm are certainly better than they are from obtaining seafood swimming in polluted lakes and seas.

HIDDEN ADDITIVES IN FISH

Sometimes fish can become a hazard because of the steps taken to prevent or cover up spoilage. Shrimp and other seafood are sometimes treated with sulfites—preservatives that can kill those allergic to them. The FDA sets limits on the residues of these chemicals in seafood and requires that their presence be revealed on the label of packed shrimp.

In the first edition of this book, I described how efforts to cover up a rotting fish product led to death. Because a three-year-old boy of Haddon Heights, New Jersey, was hungry a little earlier than usual, his mother cooked some fillet of flounder for him; the rest of the family was to eat their portion of the fish later. The little boy gobbled it down, ate his dessert, drank some milk, and then announced that he was going to his grandmother's nearby.

The rest of the family sat down to eat their dinner after the boy had left.

The child had just reached his grandmother's when he complained of feeling ill. He turned blue and began gasping for air. An ambulance was summoned, but before it could speed its tiny burden to the hospital, the little boy died.

His parents and the rest of the family, all of whom were in the midst of their meal when they heard about the boy, stopped eating. But they began to suffer from dizziness, nausea, and cyanosis (lack of oxygen).

Later that evening, the Poison Control Center in Philadelphia reported to the chief of the Philadelphia Milk and Food Sanitation Section that three women who had eaten at a Philadelphia restaurant were hospitalized when they became ill within an hour after their meal. All three women had eaten flounder. All three had become faint, suffered headaches, dizziness, and vomiting, and were cyanotic.

Robert C. Stanfill, at the time district director of the Food and Drug Administration and a neighbor of the boy's family, was shaving when he heard a report of the youngster's death on the radio. He left immediately for his office.

He and physicians and other inspectors who become involved in the case concluded that sodium nitrite, a chemical that looks like ordinary table salt but is illegally used to freshen rotting fish, was probably the cause of the poisoning. A chemist was assigned to run tests for nitrites on portions of the foods eaten by the victims.

The owner of the fish-processing firm was convicted of adding sodium nitrite to fish to cover up rottenness. He received a suspended sentence and a fine.

The amount of nitrite used as a preservative in the fish that was eaten by the little boy was enough to kill him quickly, but there is a good possibility that smaller amounts of nitrite added to fish may kill still others, more slowly. Present law permits the addition of nitrates and nitrites in concentrations of five hundred and two hundred parts, respectively, to one million parts of fish or meat. On March 3, 1971, in an article in the *Journal of Agricultural and Food Chemistry,* a publication of the American Chemical Society, five FDA chemists reported "potent cancer agents called N-nitrosamines are present in certain fish that have been treated with ordinary food preservatives consisting of nitrogen compounds called nitrates and nitrites." The chemists were Thomas Fazio, Joseph N. Damieo, John W. Howard, Richard H. White, and James O. Watts. They called the N-nitrosamines one of "the most formidable and versatile groups of carcinogens yet discovered" and said that there is a growing apprehension among experts about the use of nitrites and nitrates. N-nitrosamines are formed when nitrates and nitrites combine with amine, a chemical naturally present in the stomach (see pages 74–75).

SOLUTIONS

So what can we do about all these problems with fish—a basically delicious and nutritious food?

When I wrote the first edition of *Poisons in Your Food,* there was no mandatory inspection of fish. There still isn't, although seven seafood inspection bills are before Congress at this writing. Even the National Fisheries Institute is requesting federal inspection.

Consumption of seafood in the United States has grown dramatically, with per capita consumption up more than 20 percent in the past six years. How do the various species of fish and seafood rank in popularity in the United States?

1. Canned tuna accounts for 3.5 pounds of the more than 15 pounds of fish and seafood the average person consumes each year. That's over 20 percent of the total.

2. Shrimp's per capita consumption exceeds 2 pounds.

3. Other leading species are cod, salmon, clams, flounder, and pollock.

These seven leaders represent about 80 percent of total consumption. Other species accounting for most of the remaining 20 percent are catfish, crabs, lobsters, snapper, and trout.

Exports of U.S. fishery products now exceed $2 billion annually. The domestic and overseas growth has been fueled by physicians and nutritionists urging that fish be substituted for red meat. Nonetheless, there are growing consumer concerns over environmental pollution, new technologies, and food safety in general.[30]

There is a perception that the industry is concentrated only on the nation's coasts, but that's not accurate. There are processing plants in most states, as well as in the District of Columbia. Only a few interior states are without at least one fish processor.

There are a thousand kinds of fish, from anchovies and shrimp to tuna and swordfish, harvested from tidewater shallows to the depths of the sea. Fish have an intimate association with their environment, and water quality is not as easy to control or evaluate as is the condition of a livestock feed lot.

Currently seafood processing plants and products are monitored sporadically by a hodgepodge of agencies with overlapping jurisdictions. Fish and shellfish grown or caught in the United States are monitored by the FDA through a compliance program that requires each of the agency's twenty-one districts to obtain locally at least twelve samples a year, collected as close as possible to where the commercial catches were obtained.

The FDA inspects U.S. fish and seafood plants for compliance with sanitation and processing regulations. It also monitors fish and seafood products that are imported into the United States or are shipped interstate for compliance with the Food, Drug and Cosmetics Act. The FDA must rely almost solely on random sampling to determine safety and compliance.

The U.S. Department of Commerce operates a voluntary Fishery Products Inspection Program, which allows processors, for a fee, to have fishery products manufactured in this country inspected, graded, and certified, and imported products inspected and certified.

Fish and shellfish are among the food products subject to inspection not only by state health departments or a related agency but also by federal programs.

Finally, twenty-three coastal states whose waters produce clams, oysters, and mussels have joined with the FDA, the National Oceanic and Atmospheric Administration, and other federal agencies in a program called the Interstate Shellfish Sanitation Conference. Participants cooperatively monitor waters where shellfish grow, certify shellfish coming from safe-growing waters, and prohibit commercial shellfishing in waters that may have become polluted. This does not stop poachers from farming these waters during the night and selling the shellfish to willing, unscrupulous, or in some cases unknowing buyers.

What about fish imports?

Canada is our leading source of imports, supplying more than seven hundred million pounds annually of cod, haddock, flounder, lobster, scallops, and other fish products. Thailand is second, providing more than 214 million pounds a year, mostly of canned tuna. Third is Taiwan, shipping more than 208 million pounds annually, primarily raw tuna for packing in U.S.-operated factories in Puerto Rico and American Samoa. Other major sources supply the following amounts of seafood: Japan, 150 million pounds; Iceland, 124 million pounds; Korea, 175 million pounds; Ecuador, 147 million pounds; and Mexico, 159 million pounds.

Eighty-seven percent of the fish is not inspected,[31] and for the 13 percent that is, fish inspectors still rely mostly on their noses rather than on laboratory studies to sniff out decomposition of fish around the docks. Now, they have experienced "noses" and decomposing fish can stink, but fish with certain dangerous bacterial, parasitic, and viral infections may not.

Americans eat more than forty-three times as much beef and three times as much poultry as they do seafood, yet 24 percent of all foodborne outbreaks is due to seafood.[32]

The General Accounting Office, the "watchdog" of Congress, studied the fish situation and issued a statement in August 1988, saying that "while there is room for improvement, there does not appear to be a compelling case at this time for a comprehensive, mandatory federal seafood inspection program such as those for meat and poultry."

The GAO listed as its principal concerns the need to:

- Develop better tests to measure microbiological contamination in shellfish-growing waters and in shellfish harvests.
- Develop greater public awareness of health risks associated with eating raw or undercooked shellfish.
- Intensify efforts by state and federal law-enforcement officials to curtail illegal harvesting and distribution of shellfish from areas that are contaminated or closed to harvesting.
- Do more testing of shellfish for heavy metals and other chemical contamination.

The National Fisheries Institute (NFI), the largest seafood trade association, supports legislation to establish a federal inspection program dedicated to and specifically designed for fish and seafood. The NFI represents eleven hundred member companies involved in all aspects of the seafood industry.

At a public meeting held before the National Academy of Sciences on January 31, 1989, in Washington, D.C., Lee J. Weddig, of the NFI, said that the NFI had initiated congressional action in 1985 that directed the National Marine Fisheries Service to design an improved inspection system based on the Hazard Analysis Critical Control Point concept (HACCP). Weddig noted: "This Model Seafood Surveillance Development project has been under way during the past two years with full cooperation of the industry, which has participated in more than twenty HACCP workshops,"

Weddig said. "The project also includes a study by the National Academy of Sciences on relationships of seafood to food-borne illnesses and means of reducing such incidents."

Weddig said that NFI believes the system should include the following:

- Certification of plants. This would involve an initial inspection of facilities and procedures; in short, assurance that the facility has the capability of producing a wholesome product. The facility requirements must be specific to the type of processing and species handled.
- Surveillance of operations. Require plant operators and inspectors to verify plant adherence to HACCP procedures on an as-needed basis by the designated authority. The intensity of this surveillance would vary according to the degree of risk involved in the process and the record of the operator.
- Inspection of imports. Foreign governments wishing to have products imported into the United States would establish regulatory programs that would provide assurance of compliance with U.S. regulations. The level of sophistication in these systems would be measured by site visits and port-of-entry monitoring.
- Increased monitoring of the water in which molluscs are growing. Additional research to improve the reliability of the system is needed, as well as funding to the states for increased shellfish monitoring and enforcement.
- Toxic substance monitoring. While current levels of contamination due to industrial pollution have not had widespread impact on the safety of coastal and oceanic resources, there is a need for continual monitoring of the resources for toxic substance residues. This effort on both domestic and imported products would serve to trigger compliance efforts through the HACCP programs and port-of-entry inspections if and when the surveillance shows persistent presence of toxins at levels of concern.
- Economic violation enforcement. The inspection system should include monitoring for economic abuses and strict enforcement of labeling and packaging regulations.

Establishing a comprehensive system of this nature is challenging and complicated. NFI urges Congress to begin immediately the necessarily painstaking process in order to pass legislation:

It's obvious that the data regarding safety of seafood must be related to specific geography, species, methods of preparation to be of use. They must also be related to the source of both the fish and the contamination. It does no good to mandate regulation of commercial harvesters or processors if the source of fish that causes illness is private recreational fishing.

It is equally futile to regulate fish processors if illness is caused by mishandling fish at retail stores or in restaurants or by the consumer himself. Likewise, if problems are confined to isolated species or preparations, new regulatory needs for the vast majority of the industry may be minimal.

The relative seriousness of illnesses caused by seafood must be scrutinized. While the industry has concern over any illness caused by its products, there obviously must be a difference in intensity of regulatory efforts aimed at preventing life threatening illness versus discomfort.

The committee needs to analyze the makeup of the overall U.S. fish supply. Accepting for a moment the theory that such chemicals as PCBs, DDT, et al. as found in fish really have the potential for harm after long-term exposure, it would be useful to know what portion of the supply has any likelihood of contributing to the problem. As an example, the only commercial fish to routinely exceed the FDA tolerance for PCBs appear to be the largest bluefish. Their commercial catch amounts to 4/100's of one percent of the U.S. fish supply. How then did we get to a point of general hysteria about PCBs in fish?

The committee should also take a look at the phenomenon of burn spots, fin rot, etc. Are these really health hazards or indicators of temporary changes in the environment? Are they new or newly publicized? Of what magnitude and significance is the presence of medical waste on the shore? It is true the entire furor of the summer of 1988 was caused by a few garbage bags of waste—with little real significance other than fuel for sensational TV reports.

Finally, the committee should review the difference in standards that exist in our public health agencies.

Do the FDA and the U.S.D.A. treat the presence of salmonella in the same manner? Do they use the same criteria for determining the seriousness and regulatory posture for listeria or other microbiological organisms? Do they use analytical procedures of equal precision? Do they have the same attitudes towards reconditioning a rejected product? Do they have the same attitudes toward labeling information? . . . toward defect action levels [i.e., toward taking action against defective products]? How is it that a feed additive can be okay for poultry, but outlawed for aquaculture?[33]

While consumer groups, the fish industry, and the government are favoring the same type of inspection system for fish that exists for meat and poultry, Cornell University food scientist Joe M. Regenstein, testifying before Congress February 7, 1990, favors another type of inspection for the fish industry—continuous testing for chemical and microbial contamination.

Regenstein, a professor of food science, explained that because most seafood is harvested "in the wild," it is often affected by environmental pollution and microorganisms. "Many of the safety problems associated with seafood do not lend themselves to detection by visual checks," he pointed out.

While noting that current monitoring of shellfish beds is insufficient, he said that certain fin fish from tropical areas eat microorganisms that cause the fish to be poisonous to humans. "A system of rapid testing of each and every fish of these species from designated areas is needed," he emphasized.

Regenstein also stressed the need for expanding testing of fish growing in waters contaminated with pollutants such as PCBs, heavy metals, and pesticides. The scientific community know which species are more prone to accumulations of these pollutants and can test for their content of contaminants.[34]

When the first edition of this book came out in 1969, the same needs and remedies for fish inspection were described. Will we get mandatory fish inspection?

Weddig said in his summary:

We see an improved regulatory system combining a series of new or expanded inspection and self-monitoring efforts. The system would be mandatory, but extremely flexible in making adjustments according to actual risk associated with the type of product.

If nothing is done to protect fish in the waters and to inspect fish destined for the American dinner table, there will be fewer and fewer fish meals in the future.[35]

WHAT YOU CAN DO

How can you tell whether a fish is fresh?

In its frozen state, you can't!

When it is fresh, you should observe the following:

1. Is it of good color?
2. Does it smell? A fishy odor does not belong to fresh fish.
3. Are the eyes clear or clouded? They should be clear.
4. If you press down, do you leave an indentation in the fish? Fresh fish flesh springs up.
5. Is the skin smooth to the touch, and firm?
6. Are the gill sections clear and intact?
7. Is the tail broken? It shouldn't be.
8. Are the scales loose and lacking a sheen?

FISH HINTS

- If you still want to eat raw fish after reading this chapter—and, admittedly, sushi and sashimi can be a delicious treat—note that FDA research has shown that the hazard of parasites can be eliminated by using for raw fish dishes fish that has been properly frozen for sixty hours and then thawed.
- Keep seafoods cold. Keep fresh or smoked seafood products refrigerated at 32°F to 40°F. Thaw frozen seafoods in the refrigerator or under cold running water. Keep frozen products rigidly frozen until ready to use. Store in freezer at 0°F.

- Don't cross-contaminate. Handle raw and cooked seafood products separately; sanitize work space between preparation and serving of seafoods. Keep raw and cooked foods from coming in contact with each other.
- Know your seafood seller. Buy seafood products from approved licensed stores and markets.
- Freeze fish before preparing raw seafood dishes such as seviche, sushi, and sashimi.
- Cook fish thoroughly. Fish is cooked when it begins to flake and reaches an internal temperature of 145°F.
- Purchase raw shellfish carefully. Buy raw oysters, clams, and mussels only from approved, reputable sources. If in doubt, ask the seafood market personnel to show you the certified shipper's tag that accompanies shell stock or check the shipper number on shucked oyster containers.
- Keep "live" shellfish "alive." Don't cook or eat shellfish such as lobster, crabs, clams, oysters, or mussels if they have died during storage. Discard them.
- Refrigerate live shellfish properly. Live shellfish, such as clams, mussels, and oysters, should be stored under well-ventilated refrigeration, not in airtight plastic bags or containers. Live lobsters and crabs should also be stored in a well-ventilated area; store with damp paper towels over them in the refrigerator.
- Eat your own catch. If you catch your own fish or shellfish from local waters, make sure the waters are approved for harvest. Check with your local state department of health.
- Seafood should always be refrigerated at 43°–45°F or frozen at 0°F.
- Almost any fish can be baked, broiled, poached, steamed, or fried. Some people prefer to bake fatty fish and poach or steam lean fish. Fish fillets and steaks are excellent charcoal-broiled or barbecued.
- Allow ten minutes' cooking time for each inch of thickness at the thickest part of the fish unless the fish is less than half an inch thick. Turn it halfway through the cooking time. Fish is cooked properly when the thickest part becomes opaque and the fish flakes easily when poked with a fork.

- Bake at 450°F.
- Broil about five inches from the heat source.
- Poach in liquid at a simmer or steam on a rack over boiling liquid (covered).
- Stew in seasoned broth with cooked vegetables. Add fish at the end of the stewing time to avoid overcooking fish and undercooking vegetables.
- To microwave, check the oven manual. Generally, cook three to five minutes on high setting, being sure fish is evenly heated. Allow cooked fish to stand five to ten minutes before eating.
- Deep-fat frying adds both fat and calories. Batter-fried cod with tartar sauce and cheese on a bun can contain more fat and calories than a double cheeseburger or a quarter-pound hamburger.
- Shrimp can be simmered three to five minutes, depending on the size and quantity, or until the shells turn red. Or steam shrimp on a rack over boiling liquid ten to fifteen minutes, or sauté in margarine or butter five to ten minutes or until the flesh turns white tinged with pink.
- Steam clams and mussels over boiling water until the shells open (five to ten minutes). Oysters should be sautéed, baked, or boiled about five minutes until plump.

According to Dr. Herbert L. DuPont, professor and director of the program in infectious diseases and clinical microbiology at the University of Texas Medical School, Houston, you need four or five minutes of steaming to make the clams safe. If you cook shellfish for seven or eight minutes, they probably will be tough.

6 ⌐ Salmonella Sam and the Ptomaine Picnic

Most of us have diarrhea at one time or another, but we tend to shrug it off as a discomforting nuisance that will last only a short time. Yet, according to a study by two food safety scientists at the Food and Drug Administration, diarrheal disease is an important public health problem that is seriously underestimated and underreported. It afflicts millions of Americans—often as a direct result of the foods they eat—and it costs millions of dollars a year in lost wages and medical bills.[1] It is brought on by numerous pathogens (bacteria and viruses), many of them only recently discovered by scientists.[2]

Diarrheal disease is reaching alarming proportions among children in the nation's day-care centers, and adults who suffer sporadic episodes of diarrhea may develop long-term, debilitating diseases including rheumatoid arthritis, cardiovascular disease, and allergies.[3]

"Diarrhea is an explosive response by the body, a means of purging the gastrointestinal tract of 'unwanted, possibly harmful organisms or substances,'" Douglas L. Archer, an FDA microbiologist, explains.[4]

> When a pathogen invades the body, it can strip away the mucous layer, leaving you with no barrier of defense. That makes it easier for organisms to penetrate the absorptive cells

and destroy them, and any antibodies would be flushed out. Thus, in a sense, for a period of time, you are without the normal protection you would have against viruses.

In conditions like colitis, where the cells may have been invaded by pathogens like Shigella [see pages 166–167], damage can be produced that extends to the area where the normal immune system resides. As long as that bug is there, the normal defense mechanisms attack it, but at the same time, they are killing good cells. That is called "inflammatory bowel disease" and when that occurs, it can become a chronic inflammatory condition where you are malabsorbing and your normal defenses are thrown out of whack.

That fact is that foodborne bacteria and viruses can not only make us miserable for a period of time, they can have long-term effects or they can kill quickly.

Basing their calculations on various scientific studies and other health data, the FDA scientists—Douglas L. Archer and John E. Kvenberg—estimate that between 68.7 and 275 million cases of diarrhea occur in the United States each year. Diarrhea is a major symptom of food poisoning, and their study estimates that from 21 million to more than 81 million of all diarrhea cases are of foodborne origin, a conclusion that calls into question the food sanitation and hygienic practices followed in many homes, restaurants, and other feeding institutions. Of major concern in their study notes is diarrhea among children in day-care centers, where, by one estimate, 3,740,000 children—out of 11,000,000 enrolled—are victims of the disease annually. Another 300,000 adult employees of the centers also are afflicted each year.[5]

Archer and Kvenberg are on the staff of the division of microbiology in the FDA's Center for Food Safety and Applied Nutrition. Archer, a microbiologist who specializes in immunology, is the division's deputy director. Kvenberg, an entomologist by training, is assistant to the director and deputy program manager for the center's biological hazards program. (The authors stressed that the views expressed in the study were their own and not necessarily those of the FDA.)

Archer and Kvenberg's estimates of foodborne diarrheal disease substantially exceed previous reports by other scientists who, like the two FDA men, closely monitor the public health and economic impact infectious pathogens have on foodborne and other diseases.

"While the statement of the problem may be much lower than it really is, concern is growing over the number of pathogens (many of them newly discovered) that are causing the problem," Kvenberg said. "We're finding more and more causes of diarrhea associated with the food supply and with enteric (intestinal) pathogens, and we're finding that the population of people infected is much larger than we thought."

Why is the reporting about diarrheal diseases so uncertain?

Researchers point out that the foods are not always available for analysis, so it is hard to determine what caused the problem. Scientists don't have tests available to identify some pathogens. Only one person out of every twenty-five at best and one out of every one hundred at worst seeks medical care.

A NEWLY RECOGNIZED KILLER

In 1983, thirty-four pregnant Canadian women and/or their new-born infants became very ill. Their symptoms included blood poisoning, meningitis (inflammation of the covering of the brain), and bleeding within the womb. Seven mothers and nearly half the infants died. Two years later, on a beautiful spring day, 181 Californians began coming down with the same symptoms as the Canadian mothers and infants. Fifty of the Californians died.

What was it that caused such severe illness and so many fatalities?

It was *Listeria monocytogenes,* primarily a soilborne bacteria that had been thought of as relatively harmless to humans for more than sixty years.[6]

Raw cabbage manufactured commercially as coleslaw was incriminated in the Canadian outbreak. Investigators linked the coleslaw to the fields where the cabbage had been grown on soil contaminated by the fecal droppings from *Listeria*-stricken sheep.

Mexican-style cheese produced by a company in California caused the California outbreak of listeriosis.

Shortly after that, a well-known company had to withdraw from the United States market large quantities of ice cream owing to contamination by *L. monocytogenes.*

The immediate consequence of the cheese-borne outbreak in California was a worldwide screening of all cheeses for the possible presence of *L. monocytogenes.* The results were of great concern primarily to European cheese manufacturers who exported great quantities of their cheese to North America. The results of a year of study showed that Austrian, Danish, French, German, and Swiss cheese produced by well-known companies displayed rather frequent contamination from virulent *L. monocytogenes* on the surfaces, the rind, or crust.

Monocytogenes has been found with "frightening frequency," according to a 1988 report by H. R. Seeliger in the medical journal *Infection.*[7] He said it is in raw meat and meat products, including sausage to be consumed unheated. This may represent another important source of human contact with the organism. At least such raw meat products seem to be a greater risk to the consumer than do chickens, which have frequently been found to have *L. monocytogenes* on their surface after slaughtering. As the bodies are usually well heated before consumption, the danger is low. But the risk for spreading the organisms in the kitchen or refrigerator should not be overlooked.

With this newly recognized danger, as with most other food bacterial contaminants, *proper handling and cooking will make the item safe.* However, if it is eaten raw, as in the case of the coleslaw, or is eaten cold, as was the Mexican cheese, you have to depend on the producers to protect you.

As an added precaution, *Do not eat the rind along with the cheese. Remove it, then wash your knife, the place where you cut the cheese, and your hands.*

Listeria is a somewhat newly recognized source of foodborne disease, but one that has been well known and suffered by probably everyone reading this book more than once is *Salmonella.*

SALMONELLA

The *Salmonella* organism—named for the American veterinarian Dr. D. E. Salmon—occurs in the intestinal tract and tissues of infected humans and animals. Many of the more than twelve hundred different types can cause food poisoning. They enter the food supply through meats or animal products from infected animals or from contamination by an infected animal or person. The common symptoms are diarrhea, abdominal cramps, fever, and sometimes vomiting, which occur six to forty-eight hours after eating. Infections range from moderate, with recovery in three to four days, to fatal.

In the spring of 1985, the worst recorded epidemic of food poisoning in United States history occurred. The Hillfarm Dairy processed about 1.5 million pounds of milk a day and sold it to 217 supermarkets operated by the Jewel Food Stores chain in Illinois, Indiana, Iowa, and Michigan. The dairy, also owned by the Jewel company, had been producing milk since 1968.

The outbreak began April 9, 1985, following a scattered trickle of patients into Chicago-area hospitals and doctors' offices in late March. The cases were at first diagnosed as "the flu." The illnesses were actually caused by *Salmonella typhimurium,* one of whose characteristics is its resistance to certain antibiotics.

At least 16,285 persons are known to have been victims of the outbreak, all but 1,059 of them from Illinois. The others lived in Indiana, Iowa, Michigan, Minnesota, and Wisconsin. That is the number of culture-proven cases. There may have been many more. The organism directly caused the deaths of two persons and was a contributing factor in the deaths of four, possibly five, others.[8]

The Illinois outbreak triggered one of the most intensive investigations ever made of a milk-borne epidemic. What made it so frightening, according to the FDA, was the fact that thousands of people had become ill from drinking one of the most closely regulated products in the food supply. For years, milk has had the enviable record of being one of the nation's safest foods because it is a pasteurized product.

At most dairies, that means heating the milk to at least 161°F for at least fifteen seconds and then quickly cooling it—thus destroying microorganisms that could contaminate the milk.

Elaborate tests were done to uncover possible defects in equipment at the Hillfarm Dairy but the task force concluded that the most likely source of the outbreak was a stainless-steel pipe called a cross-connection. The pipe, about ten feet long, was linked on one side to piping that carried unpasteurized milk, and on the other to pipes carrying pasteurized skim milk. Valves at each end were supposed to prevent unpasteurized milk from mixing with the pasteurized products, and it is believed, but it is not certain, that something went wrong in the cross-connection.

A Cook County, Illinois, circuit court judge decided on January 22, 1987, that the Jewel company should not have to pay the $100 million in punitive damages sought in a class-action suit by people made ill by the contaminated milk. A jury had found that charges of "wanton and willful misconduct" by the supermarket chain in connection with the Salmonella outbreak were unfounded.

Most outbreaks of Salmonella are not so dramatic and are not even recognized. It is estimated that 1 percent of the population of the United States becomes infected each year.

In the spring of 1989, another dairy product, cheese, was linked to an outbreak of Salmonella in Minnesota, North Dakota, and Wisconsin. Health officials in Minnesota, who issued a report on January 23, 1990, said that there were 147 documented cases of salmonellosis in the three states but the health officials estimated the outbreak involved up to 15,000 cases in many other states, most of which went undetected. The outbreak was traced to a Wisconsin cheese producer's mozzarella. The contamination was detected by the Canadian Government's Health Protection Branch, where the Minnesota officials had sent samples. Canadians use a technique that is not standard in American laboratories.[9]

Eggs have been known for a long time to be the culprits in Salmonella infections. In fact, we Americans almost finished off our British allies during World War II with spray-dried eggs. We gave them twenty-two types of Salmonella they had never had before, and when Churchill referred to "blood, sweat, and tears," he may have meant more than we thought he did.[10]

The FDA is now so concerned about the continued spread of the problem of *Salmonella enteritidis*–contaminated, unbroken, Grade A shell eggs that it has recommended that all institutions discontinue use of raw, shelled eggs pooled from various sources and instead use shell eggs clearly labeled pasteurized.[11] This is especially important for nursing homes and hospitals, as the elderly and those with weakened immune systems are at high risk of serious illness if they eat eggs contaminated with *S. enteritidis,* the FDA said.

The agency said that the problem with contaminated eggs appeared to be limited to the northeastern United States. In the last two years, however, although the heaviest incidence continues to be in New England and the Middle Atlantic states, there have been a growing number of sporadic reports from the Southeast, Midwest, and West of cases of *S. enteritidis.* Recent outbreaks traceable to eggs occurred in Virginia, the District of Columbia, Illinois, and Texas.

According to the Centers for Disease Control: "Since 1979, isolation rates of *Salmonella enteritidis* [SE] infections have increased dramatically in New England and, more recently, in the mid-Atlantic states. As of October 31, 1989, 49 SE outbreaks had been reported for 1989; these outbreaks have been associated with 1,628 cases and 13 deaths. From 1985 through 1988, state health departments reported 140 SE outbreaks associated with 4,976 ill persons and 30 deaths. Contaminated food was implicated in 89 outbreaks; Grade A shell eggs were implicated in 65. From 1985 to 1989, the proportion of outbreaks from outside New England and the mid-Atlantic regions increased from 5 percent to 43 percent.[12]

The FDA is working, at the time of this writing, with local and state health departments, industry representatives, the CDC, and the Department of Agriculture to determine the best way to control these outbreaks, which result not from contamination during the cooking or storage process, but from *S. enteritidis* passed from an infected hen to the egg. Although the organism is present in the uncracked egg, thorough cooking can kill it.

Special precautions are needed when eggs are served or sold to people in high-risk categories who are particularly vulnerable to *Salmonella enteritidis* infections: the very young, the elderly, pregnant women (because of risk to the fetus), and people already weakened by serious illness or whose immune systems are weakened.

In a *Consumer Bulletin*, the United States Department of Agriculture and the Food and Drug Administration offer suggestions about how you can protect yourself and your family.

- Avoid eating raw eggs and foods containing raw eggs: homemade Caesar salad and Hollandaise sauce, for example. Products such as homemade ice cream, homemade eggnog, and homemade mayonnaise should also be avoided, but commercial forms of these products are safe to serve since they are made with pasteurized eggs. Commercial pasteurization destroys *Salmonella* bacteria.
- Cook eggs thoroughly until both the yolk and white are firm, not runny, in order to kill any bacteria that may be present. There may be some risk in eating eggs lightly cooked: soft-cooked, soft-scrambled, or sunny-side-up, for example.
- Realize that eating soft custards, meringues, French toast, and other lightly cooked foods containing eggs may also be a risk for people with weakened immune systems and other high-risk groups.
- Use Grade AA or A eggs with clean, uncracked shells. It's best if they have been stored under refrigeration.
- Refrigerate eggs at home in their original container as soon as possible, at a temperature no higher than 40°F. Do not wash eggs before storing or using them. Washing is a routine part of commercial egg processing and rewashing is unnecessary.
- Use raw shell eggs within five weeks and hard-cooked eggs (in the shell or peeled) within one week. Use leftover yolks and whites within four days.
- Avoid keeping eggs out of the refrigerator for more than two hours, including time for preparing and serving (but not cooking). If you hide hard-cooked eggs for an egg hunt, either follow the two-hour rule or do not eat the eggs.
- Wash hands, utensils, equipment, and work areas with hot, soapy water before and after they come in contact with eggs and egg-rich foods (foods with eggs as the main ingredient: quiches and baked custards, for example).

- Serve cooked eggs and egg-rich foods immediately after cooking, or refrigerate at once for serving later. Use within three to four days.
- When refrigerating a large amount of a hot egg-rich dish or leftover, divide it into several shallow containers so it will cool quickly.

HANDLING POULTRY

As you have read in chapter 4, meat and poultry are also problem carriers of *Salmonella*. Rinse all pieces thoroughly under cold, running water. After the pieces are cut up, the utensils and the cutting board should be washed in hot soapy water to prevent cross-contamination.

Salmonella resistant to antibiotics is increasing, and on page 96 you read about one of the major reasons this is occurring.

Our ability to stop *Salmonella* and the misery it causes seems almost nonexistent today. Former FDA commissioner Dr. James Goddard was quoted in the first-edition of this book as having said that one of the most dangerous sources of the disease is "Salmonella Sam." He compares him or her with "Typhoid Mary," who was an innocent carrier of that disease. Though such people are free of symptoms, they contaminate all they touch.

"Unfortunately, there appear to be a great many carriers among those who handle our food," Dr. Goddard said. "It isn't that the food industry has a peculiar attraction for Salmonella Sams. Rather, food handlers have a greater exposure to infection because of the presence of salmonella in the food-processing environment."[13]

THE MOST COMMON BUT UNHERALDED BUG IN FOOD

Salmonellosis is considered to be a leading cause of food poisoning, but there is growing evidence that a lesser known and less publicized "bug," *Campylobacter jejuni,* is probably responsible for up to two and a half times more food-poisoning outbreaks than is *Salmonella*. If the basic data from various studies were extrapolated nationally, it would mean that approximately 2,867,000 cases of campylobacterosis occur in the United States in a year. And if similar estimates were made just for *Salmonella, Campylobacter,* and *Shigella* together, this would mean more than 4.45 million cases of diarrhea each year resulted from those three pathogens alone.

Campylobacter jejuni is a rod-shaped bacteria found in poultry, cattle, and sheep and can contaminate the meat and milk of these animals. Chief food sources are raw poultry and meat and unpasteurized milk. The onset of symptoms—diarrhea, abdominal cramping, fever, and sometimes bloody stools—is generally two to five days after eating. A Seattle–King County surveillance study of campylobacteriosis found that the total length of illness was greater for *C. jejuni* patients than for salmonellosis patients. The average length of illness for campylobacteriosis was 13.52 days to 14.2 days, while the average length of illness for salmonellosis was 10.25 days to 5.82 days.[14]

BOTULISM

The toxin responsible for botulism is the most powerful and deadly poison known to man. Cobra venom, curare, and arsenic are mild by comparison. Controlled experiments at the University of Michigan have shown that one-trillionth part of a gram of pure botulism toxin is enough to kill an adult. It is so potent, it has long been recognized as a prospective weapon for biological warfare.[15]

Botulism was first recorded as a disease in 1735, in Germany. At the time, the poisoning appeared to be associated with sausage, and the disease was named "botulinus" from the Latin word for "sausage," *botulus.* Not until 1895 was the organism discovered and described as occurring in ham and pork. It was called Type A. Thirty years later, a second type, named B, was found in California soil. Since then, it has been found in soils all over the world. Types A and B are both often associated with vegetables and fruit.

In subsequent years, two more types were discovered, C and D. Type C was found to occur in birds and has, periodically, created havoc in the population of wild ducks. According to Professor Elizabeth McCoy, of the University of Wisconsin, no human case of Type C has yet been authentically reported.

Type D was found to be associated with diseases of grazing animals—horses, cattle, sheep—and has been called "forage poisoning." Animals pick it up by feeding on decomposed vegetation that often contains the growing bacteria. This type, like C, also appears incapable of affecting human beings.

The last type found to date, Type E, was discovered in saltwater fish. Poisoning from it occurs most frequently in countries where much preserved fish is consumed. It wasn't until 1951 that scientists discovered that Type E could also come from freshwater fish.[16]

The largest outbreak of botulism ever recorded occurred in Russia in 1933. Some 230 cases, with 94 deaths, resulted from Type A toxin present in stuffed eggplant.

The victims of botulism usually get it by eating improperly canned foods—meat, fish, or nonacid vegetables. Once in the body, the toxin is absorbed sluggishly by the intestines. But when it gets into the bloodstream, the consequences are swift. The poison sets up roadblocks between nerves and muscles, causing paralysis. Breathing muscles are usually the first to suffer, then the heart muscle.

Take the case of the lethal lunch described in the first edition of *Poisons in Your Food*:

While the two Detroit women talked, Helen Brown took some salad dressing she had made and mixed it with the tuna fish.

"That fish smells kind of funny," Barbara Mason said, picking up the can and sniffing it. "Do you smell anything?"

"No, it smells all right to me. Let me taste some," Helen replied. "It tastes all right!"

She finished making the sandwiches and then decided to open a can of soup because it was such a chilly day. They were almost through with lunch when Mrs. Brown's mother, Mrs. Konners, dropped in.

"Hi, Mother," Helen said. "Why don't you have some lunch with us?"

"I'm not very hungry," Mrs. Konners replied, "but I'll take a taste of that tuna fish. I want to see if you made it as good as I make it."

The three chatted for a while until it was time for the children to return from school.

That night at dinner—about 6:00 P.M.—Helen Brown complained to her husband that her vision was blurred. She kept taking off her glasses and putting them on again. Without finishing the dishes after supper, she went to bed.

"It's hard to breathe," she told her husband, "and my throat feels tight."

She and her husband thought she was coming down with the flu. They believed she would be all right in the morning.

But at 6:30 A.M., Mr. Brown was awakened by the sounds his wife was making. She was breathing convulsively and could speak only in a whisper. He called the emergency squad, and his wife was taken to the hospital. But before the ambulance arrived, at 7:30 A.M., Helen Brown was dead.

Her luncheon companion, Barbara Mason, had also begun to feel the same symptoms around dinnertime on the day of the lunch. She complained of dizziness and of blurred vision, and had difficulty breathing. Later, her movements became somewhat uncoordinated, and she vomited frequently during the night. She and her husband both thought it was the flu until they heard about Helen Brown.

Barbara Mason was hospitalized half an hour after her friend's death. She was given polyvalent Types A and B botulinus antitoxin. Her symptoms continued to progress. On the fourth day after the luncheon, she was given Type E antitoxin. She did not improve. At 5:00 P.M., five days after the fateful lunch, Barbara Mason joined her friend in death.

Helen Brown's mother, Mrs. Konners, did not suffer the symptoms until about twenty-four hours after eating a small portion of tuna salad. She began vomiting and also complained of a sore throat and some difficulty with her vision. She was hospitalized and given ten thousand units of A and B polyvalent botulinus antitoxin. Her recovery was relatively rapid and she was released from the hospital three days later.

Laboratory tests confirmed that the illness that struck the three women was botulism.

Samples from Mrs. Brown's garbage can, including some of the salad dressing, the soup can, and the tuna can, were given to the public health laboratory. Even the can opener was brought in. A pure culture of botulinus was isolated from the tuna can.

The state health department of Michigan, the Wayne County, Michigan, Health Department, the Detroit district of the federal Food and Drug Administration and the California State Health Department immediately began tracking down cans from the same lot of tuna fish. The California State Department of Health closed down the cannery that packed the tuna. The tuna fish had been imported frozen from Japan and canned in the California plant.

On the same day the plant was closed down, the New York City Health Department picked up a large number of cans in that city. In all, health officials retrieved twelve hundred cans. Tests showed that at least twenty-one contained the deadly botulinus.[17]

This was the first incident of botulism arising from commercially canned foods in the United States in nearly forty years. One exception may be a reported incident, caused by commercially canned mushroom sauce, which occurred in 1941. The United States canning industry has maintained a good record for safety.

In 1963, the same year as the deaths from poisonous tuna fish, nineteen more cases of botulism were reported as being caused by commercially smoked fish. Seven persons died. In the same year, home-processed foods were responsible for twenty-two cases of botulism, including five deaths.[18]

On June 30, 1971, a New York banker and his wife shared a can of Bon Vivant vichyssoise soup. The man was dead within a few hours after the meal. His wife was paralyzed. Their blood tests showed botulism poisoning, and so did the remaining soup in the can.[19]

The company that made the soup, Bon Vivant, produced vichyssoise under twenty-two brands. Thanks to quick work by the FDA and the cooperation of the press and merchants, no other cases of botulism were reported. The company, however, did not survive the publicity.

In 1989, two men and a woman in Kingston, New York, came down with botulism after eating garlic bread made with a garlic-and-oil mix. That year the FDA recommended that homemade and commercial garlic-and-oil products that do not have antimicrobial agents be discarded.[20] There were no preservatives in the oil, according to the FDA, and the agency cautioned that such prepared garlic should have antimicrobials and also be refrigerated.

In 1989, there was also an outbreak of botulism in fish prepared Russian style, in New York (see page 134).

But no one knows how many cases of botulism there really are each year.

An editorial in the *Journal of the American Medical Association* pointed out that because of the relative rarity of botulism, "the diagnosis would not be in the front of the physician's mind and botulism could be overlooked."[21]

"During publicized epidemics, every news reader will know as much about botulism as the physician," the editorial said. "How many physicians know that they can obtain types A and B antitoxin from ready commercial sources and Type E from the Public Health Service Communicable Disease Center in Atlanta, which began to stockpile significant quantities more than a year ago?"

The fear that botulism may again become a threat is based on the new method of selling food *sous-vide,* or vacuum-packaged and partially cooked (see pages 133–134).

THE PTOMAINE PICNIC

Foodborne illness from *Staphylococcus* is often referred to by laymen as "ptomaine" poisoning. This term has been consistently used since its introduction in 1870. Actually, there is no specific entity or group of substances that properly might be called "ptomaine." *Staphylococcus* is derived from the Greek word *staphylo,* which means "a bunch of grapes," and *coccus,* which means "carcass" or "dead flesh." The *Staphylococcus* bacteria often looks like a bunch of grapes.

Staphylococci are often called "opportunists" because they wait for suitable conditions to invade the body. Staph is present on human skin, in the human throat, and in the human nasal areas, as well as in festering human wounds. Food handlers with staphylococcal skin infections are the primary source of the illness.

Many foods, once infected, will allow the organisms to grow and produce toxins unless the food is refrigerated. Even if the organism itself has been killed by heat, if sufficient toxin has been produced the food is still capable of causing the symptoms of staph poisoning. The toxin produced by staph is heat-resistant.

The foods most often connected with staph poisoning are cus-tards, cream-filled pastry, milk, and processed meat and fish. For some odd reason, these *staphylococci* seem to love church affairs. At one church dinner, for example, over half of those who had eaten chicken—about one hundred persons—became ill within six hours. The chickens had been cooked the day before and immediately refrigerated. The next morning, they were reheated and cut into quarters with a butcher's meat saw. The chickens were without refrigeration from 10:00 A.M. until 5:00 P.M., when they were again reheated. The hands of the cook who prepared the chickens had numerous small cuts and abrasions.

The incubation period is usually two to four hours after ingestion of food containing enterotoxin, or "poison." Then the onset is abrupt, with nausea and vomiting. The attack lasts from three to six hours, which is too long if you've ever had it. Fatalities are rare, and complete recovery is the norm. Diagnosis is usually based on the sudden onset of illness after eating infected food, brevity of symp-toms, and rapidity of recovery. Furthermore, the patient is usually one of a number of similarly affected victims.

In the past few years, considerable progress has been made in the laboratory concerning the procedures for detecting staph poisons in food. In fact, new laboratory techniques saved a cheese manufactur-er from financial ruin. Staphylotoxin was discovered in samples of four million pounds of cheese that had been distributed around the country. Even though the live staph germ itself was not present, the cheese was ordered removed from the market. Faced with bank-ruptcy, the manufacturer had the cheese tested for the presence of enterotoxin, using the new laboratory techniques. As a result, he was able to release all but approximately sixty-two thousand pounds of the cheese. No report of food poisoning followed the consump-tion of the released cheese.

SHIGELLA

Anyone who bet on the Minnesota Vikings–Miami Dolphins October 2, 1988, game in Miami couldn't have known that the

Vikings would be overpowered by a tiny group of rod-shaped bacteria, *Shigellae*.

The *Shigellae* are, with rare exceptions, found only in the intestinal tract of man and captive monkeys. They are named after K. Shiga, a Japanese bacteriologist who first isolated a *Shigella* organism ninety years before that fateful game. In humans, *Shigellae* can cause a serious illness called shigellosis or bacillary dysentery. While shigellosis is not as common as other foodborne illnesses, large outbreaks have been reported; but with shigellosis, as with other foodborne diseases, the true incidence is greatly underreported.

The incubation period is one to four days. This is one reason that diagnosis is frequently erroneous. Suspect food after that length of time is often not available for examination. Another reason is that laboratories often fail to use techniques that will detect a small number of *Shigellae* in the presence of a larger number of other bacteria.

The trouble with the Vikings *Shigella* outbreak first came to light when twenty-one members of the football team began complaining of cramps, fever, chills, and diarrhea after taking a Northwest Airlines flight from Minneapolis to Miami. They lost the game, naturally, but they won the attention of the FDA investigators.[22]

Over the next six weeks, scores of other Northwest passengers suffered the same symptoms, setting off an intensive investigation by local, state, and federal agencies, including the FDA, which is responsible for sanitation on interstate public transportation.

Investigators tracked down over a thousand passengers from 253 Northwest flights that traveled through Minneapolis to four countries, twenty-eight states, and the District of Columbia. Seven hundred and twenty-five passengers were interviewed to determine if those who had eaten food served on the planes had become ill after their flights. Researchers also contacted another 589 Northwest passengers who had not reported becoming ill to establish a control group for their study. Interviews showed a pattern to the illness that indicated the potential for at least one thousand to twenty-five hundred cases of food poisoning and contamination of as many as 43,100 meals.

Tests of the victims' stool samples showed the culprit was *Shigella sonnei.*

Investigation into the food-poisoning outbreak traced the source of contamination to the Marriott Corporation's in-flight kitchen at the Minneapolis–St. Paul International Airport. Investigators from the FDA and Minnesota county and state health departments inspected the kitchen's food-handling and storage facilities, interviewed food handlers, and took samples of raw and prepared food for laboratory analysis.

Health records were screened to see if any employees had been ill during the outbreak, and all production employees who worked in food preparation during the outbreak were given physical examinations and blood tests.

No major sanitation problems were found.

Ironically, it was concluded that the "hero" sandwiches probably felled the Vikings. Two of the five food handlers working the shift that made the sandwiches had elevated antibodies suggesting recent *Shigella* infection.

Shigella infections are usually spread by contaminated water, defective plumbing, or food contaminated by unwashed hands or by flies. Shigellosis affects many institutionalized patients and has become resistant to antibiotics. Good sanitation, with the exclusion of flies and protection of food from contamination, is of prime importance in preventing the infection.

CLOSTRIDIUM PERFRINGENS

One day, an exclusive girls' school had almost 100 percent illness. From the headmistress to the youngest student, everyone was crowding the bathrooms with diarrhea and coliclike cramps. The suspect meal was roast beef and gravy. The beef and gravy had been prepared the day before and allowed to cool in open trays, without refrigeration, for twenty-two hours.

This type of foodborne disease has been known since 1898. By the 1950s, outbreaks resulting from *perfringens* contamination were being reported frequently in the United States and Europe. Not until recently has it been recognized as a leading cause of foodborne illness, because only recently have outbreak foods been examined for organisms that grow in the absence of air.

Clostridium perfringens is widely distributed in feces, sewage, and soil. It is so prevalent it is a probable contaminant of nearly all foods. The spores of *C. perfringens* are present in a large percentage of meat products, both raw and cooked. The cooked foods most frequently associated with outbreaks in America are meats, fowl, and gravies that have been cooked and allowed to cool slowly.

It is a rod-shaped bacterium widely distributed in nature. It is found in soil, dust, food, and the intestinal tracts of humans and other warm-blooded animals. It grows only in the absence of air (anaerobically), and when it grows it produces resistant forms called spores. It grows poorly below 70°F (21°C). However, the spores, which contain the fertile part of the organisms in a protective wall, are not injured by cold temperatures. The bacterium grows rapidly at the temperatures in the range of 85°–115°F (30°–46°F). It is killed by exposure to temperatures of 125°F (52°C) and above, but the spores are not injured until the temperature approaches that of boiling water.

Again, as with other food-poisoning organisms, good sanitary practices in the handling, preparing, and serving of foods, especially meats, gravies, and meat dishes, will help prevent illness. Meats should be cooked, kept hot, above 125°F or 52°C, and served hot.

What You Can Do at Home to Prevent *Clostridium perfringens*

- If cooked for later use, meats, gravies, and meat dishes should be cooled rapidly in small lots in the refrigerator to 45°F (7°C) or below.
- Leftover meat or meat dishes should receive adequate heat treatment before being used, and leftover gravy should be brought to a rolling boil before being served again.
- Cold cuts and cold sliced meats should be maintained cold (below 45°F or 7°C) and served cold, not at room temperature.

ESCHERICHIA COLI

As Christmas lights were being hung along the streets and while carols poured from loudspeakers in December 1965, babies began to sicken and die in Newark, New Jersey. The infants had severe diarrhea, a condition that does kill millions of infants in underdeveloped countries around the world every year. But what had caused it in New Jersey's largest city? What did the babies have in common? They came from families of all economic levels and from all ethnic groups.

By the time officials realized it was an epidemic, sickness had struck scores of babies. Public health officials who began investigating the case found that there was one thing 30 percent of the babies did have in common. They had been hospitalized in the recent past, but for a variety of conditions. Without knowing what was causing the sickness, doctors tried desperately to save the infants. They used a wide spectrum of antibiotics, but none seemed of much use.

By the time the epidemic had ended, four hundred infants had been seriously affected and twenty-eight had died. Of those that succumbed, almost all had been in the 30 percent previously hospitalized for other conditions.

Laboratories finally succeeded in isolating the organism that had caused the diarrhea. It was *Escherichia coli*.[23]

Escherichia coli are a type of short, plump, rod-shaped bacteria commonly present in the intestinal tract of humans and other warm-blooded animals and consequently in sewage and polluted waters. They are named after Dr. Escherich, a German microbiologist, who first isolated them in 1885. They are associated particularly with infant diarrhea in this country. The symptoms range from those of a mild disease to a severe illness with high fever, acute diarrhea, and prostration. In addition to the overt illness caused by ingesting *Escherichia coli,* both the acutely ill and those displaying no symptoms become carriers for variable periods of time and are potentially dangerous to small infants.

Although they are not sure, public health officials believe that the Newark infants picked up the disease in hospitals, either from food or personnel, during their stay for treatment of other conditions; then they spread the disease to other infants in the community.

Escherichia coli are important because their presence in food and water indicates contamination with fecal material. While normal *E. coli* are not in themselves considered hazardous by health officials, their presence in food or water is regarded as a warning that other more dangerous bacteria frequently found in fecal material may also be present. Food or water contaminated with fecal material may cause serious epidemics. Therefore, health officials condemn water supplies, finished foods, and any raw material contaminated with *E. coli*. They also close the beaches when *E. coli* reaches a certain level in the swimming water.

Now, it has been discovered that a new *E. coli* is very dangerous to human health.

Steve Ostroff, M.D., medical epidemiologist, Enteric Division Branch of the Centers for Disease Control in Atlanta, said the new bacteria is *E. coli 0157H7 (or Hemorrhagic E. coli)*. It was first diagnosed in 1982 in Washington and has been discovered in Canada and Great Britain.[24]

"To the best of our knowledge, it is related to dairy cattle—raw milk and ground beef consumption," he said. "People who get it get very severe bloody diarrhea, severe abdominal cramps, nausea, vomiting, and a low fever three to four days after eating contaminated food. We never had an outbreak that we knew of until it was identified in a fast-food place in Oregon. Forty percent of the victims had to be hospitalized.

"It may also have long-term consequences. It may shut down kidneys, burst red blood cells. In adults, it may cause nervous-system problems such as strokes and seizures due to blood clots in the brain."

How much of our food is contaminated with the organism? How many of our illnesses are caused by *E. coli?* Although proper laboratory tests could tell us, no one knows. *E. coli* is most commonly found in food served in public places, according to the Centers for Disease Control.

Heat and pasteurization kill the bacteria in food products. Chemicals can also destroy the organisms. However, the use of a chemical in each food product must conform to FDA regulations. Living *E. coli* on equipment can be destroyed by proper use of sanitizing compounds after hot water and detergent scrubbing and rinsing.

Even though the organisms can be killed or washed away, keeping them out of food is the best way to prevent contamination. This can be accomplished only by following good sanitation practices when preparing, processing, packaging, storing, or otherwise handling food products.

What You Can Do at Home to Prevent *E. coli* Illness

- Drink only pasteurized milk.
- After shopping, quickly freeze or refrigerate perishable foods.
- Use refrigerated ground meat and patties in three to four days, frozen meat and patties in three to four months.
- Wash your hands, utensils, and work areas with hot, soapy water after contact with raw meat and meat patties.
- Cook meat and patties until very hot. The center should be gray or brown. Juices should run clear with no trace of pink. All meat, poultry, and fish should be well cooked.
- Serve cooked food with clean plates and utensils, not ones that have been used for the raw meat.
- Check package directions. You might need to preheat the oven or grill. Cook for the required time period. Cook covered if directions call for that.
- Microwave carefully. If your oven is a lower wattage than what is shown in the instructions, you'll need to cook food longer or at a higher setting. Rotate food for even cooking. Let food stand outside the oven after cooking if that's what the directions say. The food will finish cooking as it stands.
- Never thaw food on the counter or let it sit out of the refrigerator for more than two hours.

NO BROWNIE POINTS FOR *YERSINIA ENTEROCOLITICA*

A Brownie troop leader was entertaining the group of young Girl-Scouts-to-be in her home. She wanted to serve them a healthy meal, so she prepared bean sprouts. Not long after eating the meal, the youngsters began to have stomach cramps with diarrhea and a fever. Some parents even thought their children had appendicitis.

The outbreak was traced to contaminated well water in which the bean sprouts had been placed. The children recovered, but older patients who suffer from *Yersinia* may not be so lucky. Postinfection problems may include arthritis and a red, painful rash. *Yersinia enterocolitica* is rapidly emerging worldwide as a stomach bacteria associated with a wide spectrum of clinical and immunologic manifestations. The clinical illness caused by this pathogen ranges from self-limited intestinal "upsets" to fatal systemic infections.[25]

In the past twenty years, there has been a dramatic increase in the frequency of the isolation of this organism. In several countries, including the Netherlands, Belgium, Canada, and Australia, *Y. enterocolitica* has surpassed *Shigella* and rivals *Salmonella* and *Campylobacter* as a cause of acute stomach upsets caused by bacteria.[26]

GIARDIASIS

The *Giardia* protozoa (tiny animals) exist in the intestinal tract of humans and are found in cysts that are expelled in feces. Infestation with *Giardia,* giardiasis, is most frequently associated with the consumption of contaminated water (see pages 196–197). It may, however, be transmitted by uncooked foods that become contaminated during growth or after being handled and cooked by persons infected with the organisms. Cool, moist conditions favor survival of the organism. Waterborne epidemics involving remote streams, well water, and chlorinated community systems have all been implicated. Both humans and wild animals may serve as reservoirs. The infection is found worldwide, especially in areas of poor sanitation and in children. As many as half the children in day-care centers may have giardiasis. It is also common in male homosexuals and in persons with immune deficiencies.[27]

There may be no symptoms, or the infection can manifest itself in bouts of diarrhea—or occasionally constipation—abdominal pain, intestinal gas, abdominal distention, digestive disturbances, loss of appetite, nausea, and vomiting.

Good sanitation, of course, can help prevent infection, but as a wise precaution, don't drink from mountain streams. They may look clean, but . . .

FOODBORNE ILLNESSES FROM VIRUSES

A kitchen worker in a hospital in St. Louis, Missouri, went about her duties although she was worried about her husband. He didn't complain much, but he acted as if he didn't feel too well. The date was July 2. As she mixed the frozen orange-juice concentrate with water for the next morning's breakfast, she was glad she was well and able to hold down a job to supplement the family's income. She placed the orange juice in the refrigerator and went home.

The next morning, interns, resident physicians, nurses, and cafeteria employees filed in for breakfast. Most of them, as is the custom in America, took orange juice.

Between July 21 and August 12, fourteen of the orange-juice drinkers came down with hepatitis. This was in spite of the fact that the orange juice had a pH (acidity-alkalinity content) in the range of 3.5 to 4.0 and had been left in the refrigerator at least overnight. At the time the hospital personnel came down with hepatitis, so did the kitchen worker's husband. The public health officials believe that he had the virus and that his wife carried it without symptoms.

For some reason, young people seem to be affected most frequently by hepatitis. The peak season apparently is in the fall. The incubation period for hepatitis is estimated at two to six weeks.[28] The onset of the symptoms is abrupt, with loss of appetite, nausea, fever, and malaise. Tenderness and enlargement of the liver and pain in the right upper quadrant are usually early symptoms. About five days after the onset, jaundice appears, and fever tends to subside. The gastrointestinal symptoms persist for about ten days and subside with regression of the jaundice. Swollen glands, severe generalized itching, hives, and intermittent diarrhea may occur. Usually, the patient recovers uneventfully after six to eight weeks. Relapses occur in 5 to 15 percent of the cases and are usually attributed to premature resumption of activity, poor diet, or alcoholism. Ninety percent of the patients recover.

Since the incubation period for hepatitis is approximately four weeks, it is extremely difficult to compile definitive information once an outbreak has been recognized.

Viruses are less likely to survive in foods that are well cooked.

The majority of foods implicated in the outbreaks of hepatitis had been cooked very little. However, if the contamination takes place almost immediately before the food is eaten, cooking longer may not kill the virus. As a result, the infected human who works either as a food handler or a kitchen worker in the final preparations of the meal constitutes a significant risk of contaminating the food with the virus.

As with the spread of bacteria-borne food poisoning, good sanitation is one step in prevention. As far as the hepatitis virus is concerned, public health officials agree that the virus is shed by infected individuals in the feces, so that considerable mishandling of food must occur before there is a foodborne outbreak.

TOXOPLASMOSIS

With the influx of immigrants from Third World countries and Americans' love of exotic foods, the chances of picking up parasites in food increases. Tapeworms, protozoa, and other parasites can cause all sorts of symptoms, from ulcers to weight loss to dysentery.

One foodborne disease that can cause havoc, especially with fetuses, is toxoplasmosis. An editorial in the February 4, 1988, *New England Journal of Medicine* said the tragedy of toxoplasmosis as a cause of blindness or near-blindness or of psychomotor or mental retardation in children is the fact that it can be prevented and that it has "never concerned the medical community" in the United States as it has in Europe.[29]

Toxoplasma gondii has a worldwide distribution. The prevalence of the chronic (latent) infection can vary markedly among adults, according to the *Journal,* and up to 90 percent are infected in Paris and up to 50 percent are infected in the United States. Almost all have no symptoms and will never be troubled by their infection. On the other hand, millions of dollars are needed each year to care for victims of congenital toxoplasmosis in the United States. Patients with AIDS may have clinically severe toxoplasmosis.

Toxoplasma is spread in nature by ingestion of oocysts or of tissue cysts in undercooked meat and by congenital transmission.

Oocysts are excreted in the feces of cats, the definitive hosts in nature. Ingestion of oocysts or tissue cysts results in the liberation of organisms that invade the intestinal mucosa and are then disseminated widely.

Congenital toxoplasma infections occur when the organisms infect the placenta and, after a lag period, the fetus.

Prevention of the congenital infection is achieved by preventing material infection during pregnancy and by detecting acute infection during pregnancy and treating the mother.

What You Can Do to Prevent Toxoplasmosis

- Cook meat until it is well done.
- Wash fruits and vegetables.
- Wear gloves while working in the garden or disposing of cat litter (if such handling cannot be avoided).

OTHER FOODBORNE DISEASES

There are many other foodborne diseases. In fact, more than 40 percent of all human diseases are contracted through food.

Typhoid fever, although it crops up once in a while, is not too much of a problem in America today. It can still be a danger in water, milk, and shellfish contaminated at the source. Food contaminated by unwashed hands or by flies may still give a person typhoid fever.

Streptococcus, which causes septic sore throat and scarlet fever, may still be ingested in raw milk contaminated at the source. Diphtheria is a remote danger from dishes or silverware contaminated by a carrier.

Brucellosis, or undulant fever, is an infectious disease with an acute high fever but few other signs. Vague body aches, weakness, and sweating may also be associated with it. Brucellosis can be prevented by drinking only pasteurized milk and eating aged cheese. Though brucellosis is a worldwide disease, it is most prevalent in rural areas and is an occupational disease among meat packers, veterinarians, farmers, and livestock producers.[30]

WHAT YOU CAN DO IN GENERAL

As you can see from the foodborne illnesses described above, you can prevent most of them by:

- Shopping at a store where the hygiene is good (see chapter 9).
- Cooking properly. The day of rare or uncooked meat or fish should be past unless you are in perfect health and you are the type that likes to play Russian roulette.
- Proper temperature control on your part, from the store to your home to the table, is vital (see pages 243–244).
- Good hygiene. Clean cutting boards, knives, plates, and silverware as well as clean hands can go far in preventing foodborne illnesses.

If you should become ill, proper medical attention and responsible reporting will help prevent future illness in yourself and others.

7 ～ Water: Unfit for Drinking?

A young mother leaned over the bathtub in her Lodi, New Jersey, home and turned on the water. Her four-year-old daughter giggled. The mother frowned and stared at the rushing water.

In ten seconds she found what she was looking for.

"See? There. There's one. There's another."

Floating in her white ceramic bathtub were three colorless worms, each no bigger than a fingernail clipping.

The mother was outraged at finding more than a dozen worms, some of them dark and wiggling with life, in her household's water.

The Passaic Valley Water Commission members told her and others with the same problem that the worms were actually larvae of midge flies. Aesthetically unpleasing, but not a health hazard. To prove it, the water commission's chief engineer appeared on TV and drank a bottle of wormy water.[1]

In Woburn, Massachusetts, the problem was invisible to the naked eye but far more lethal to the body. A typical old New England industrial town, Woburn is about twelve miles north of Boston. For more than 130 years, most of its workers were employed in factories. They processed leather, manufactured arsenic pesticides, and produced chemicals, textiles, paper, TNT, and animal glues.

A frightening number of children in this town of thirty-seven thousand began suffering from leukemia. Babies were being born with defects and dying shortly after birth.[2] A citizens' group—not a government agency—formed, and in late 1979 produced a list of local children diagnosed with leukemia.

Investigators from the Massachusetts Department of Public Health and the Communicable Disease Centers reviewed the death statistics from 1969 to 1979 and, indeed, found that the *overall* cancer death rate in Woburn was significantly higher than that of the state and six adjacent communities. Another investigation discovered a concentration of adult kidney cancer. The investigations concluded that there was a significantly elevated rate of childhood leukemia in Woburn between 1969 and 1979, with 12 cases diagnosed when only 5.3 were expected.

The town's drinking water was supplied by eight municipal wells, two of which—G and H—were operated as a single source in eastern Woburn. The chance discovery of some toxic wastes near the two wells led to testing their water in May 1979. The investigators looked for 32 volatile organics on the Environmental Protection Agency's list of 129 priority (dangerous) pollutants.

High levels of the solvents trichloroethylene, tetrachloroethylene, and chloroform—all potential cancer-causing agents—were detected and the wells were shut down.

The remaining town wells were tested and found to meet both state and federal drinking-water standards.

Independently, during site excavations in July 1979 for an industrial complex located north of wells G and H, large pits of buried animal hides and chemical wastes were discovered. A nearby abandoned lagoon was found to be heavily contaminated with lead, arsenic, and other metals. Subsequently, the groundwater under eastern Woburn was sampled at sixty-one test wells and found to contain forty-eight EPA priority pollutants and raised levels of twenty-two metals.

Professors S. W. Lagakos and M. Zelen and research assistant B. J. Wessen, from the department of biostatistics, Harvard School of Public Health, began their own investigation. They obtained information on twenty cases of childhood leukemia diagnosed in Woburn between 1964—the year the wells G and H began pumping—and 1983. Overall, fifteen of the twenty cases were males, seventeen had acute lymphocytic leukemia, and fifteen were born in Woburn. The median age at diagnosis was seven years.

Using interviews and painstaking research, they gathered information about the sick children and about the space-time distribution of water from the two contaminated wells. The Harvard researchers concluded that there existed "positive statistical associations between access to this water and the incidence rates of childhood leukemia, perinatal deaths (1970–1982), and some birth defects and childhood disorders.

"A key question among citizens is whether individuals who were formerly exposed to wells G and H might still be at an elevated risk," the Harvard researchers wrote in the September 1986 issue of the *Journal of the American Statistical Association.* "One way this can be investigated is by monitoring adverse health outcomes in Woburn over the next few years."

They reported that in the three years following the closure of wells G and H, the rates of perinatal deaths, birth defects, and central nervous system disorders declined to levels comparable with those of the rest of Woburn.

"If these rates, as well as those of leukemia, lung, and kidney disorders continue to remain low in these areas, individuals who were formerly exposed to wells G and H will have reason to believe that any earlier elevation in risk that might have been due to wells G and H is no longer present."[3]

Woburn is not the only town to have a correlation between chemical pollution in water and illness. Four small industrial communities in northern New Jersey with histories of chemically contaminated groundwater showed elevated levels of leukemia among women and girls from 1979 to 1984.[4] The chemicals found in the wells were industrial solvents used in dry cleaning and metal degreasing. They included trichloroethylene, tetrachloroethylene, 1,1,1-trichloroethane (TCA), and dichloroethylenes.

A health department study said that the detected levels of the four solvents in the communities ranged from 37 ppb (parts per billion) to 72 ppb. The New Jersey Department of Environmental Protection has proposed setting 30 ppb as the acceptable level. New Jersey Health Department officials said that the leukemia rate could not definitely be tied to the pollutants.

In November 1981, a leak of solvents from an underground storage tank at an electronics manufacturing plant in Santa Clara County, California, polluted well water. The solvents were predominantly 1,1,1-trichloroethane (TCA) and methyl chloroform. At the request of worried residents, the California Health Department conducted two epidemiological studies. The studies found an increased prevalence of heart defects among babies born in Santa Clara County between 1981 and 1983.

"There was a cluster [of heart defects] and there was some evidence found that case mothers were somewhat more likely to have had TCA exposure from their drinking water than control mothers at a time period in gestation critical for cardiac development," the California investigators concluded. But they too were reluctant to conclude that a definite link between the polluted well water and the birth defects existed.

INDUSTRIAL AND HOUSEHOLD CHEMICAL WASTES

The problem with contamination of water by industrial wastes is not just a Massachusetts, New Jersey, or California problem: it is nationwide.

Industrial waste pits, ponds, and lagoons are "one of the largest threats to goundwater," according to a congressional committee report.[5] Based on a survey by the U.S. Environmental Protection Agency, it is estimated that throughout the nation fifty billion gallons of liquid industrial wastes are placed in surface ponds or lagoons each day.

More than one-third of the twenty-six thousand industrial waste sites surveyed were found to be unlined; there were no barriers to prevent contaminants from seeping into the ground. Moreover, seventy-eight hundred of the unlined industrial waste lagoons were "directly on top of ground water sources, with no barrier reported between the wastes and the ground water."

Nationwide, the EPA report showed that 9.6 billion pounds of toxic chemicals were released into streams and waterways, while 1.9 billion pounds went into municipal sewer systems, 2.7 billion went into the air, and 2.5 billion onto the land. In addition, 3.2 billion pounds were injected into underground wells and 2.6 billion were sent to off-site treatment and disposal facilities.[6]

The results of such careless waste disposal can affect many people directly. For example:

California public health officials closed thirty-nine public wells supplying drinking water to more than four-hundred thousand people in the San Gabriel Valley in January 1980 because of chemical contamination. The contaminated wells were near major industrial areas.

Chem-Dyne dump in Hamilton, Ohio, was once the final dump for chemical wastes from at least 289 factories, almost every source east of the Mississippi River. In August 1982, when the U.S. Environmental Protection Agency filed suit against the owners of the defunct company and sixteen companies that disposed of wastes at the site, the dump still contained some ten thousand drums and 150,000 gallons of hazardous material. No one knows how much toxic waste was deposited there over the years.

The Chem-Dyne site sits atop the underground aquifer from which Hamilton draws its well water. Harry Marks, professor of chemistry at the University of Cincinnati, was appointed by the state of Ohio to inventory the site. Said Marks in 1982: "I would not drink the water. There is no way of knowing what's in the drinking water without very sophisticated tests. . . . The leakages were atrocious. I've been a chemist for 25 years and I've seen nothing like it. I was appalled at what was going on right in the middle of the city."[7]

STATISTICS

These cases add to the mounting evidence that we all have a big problem with toxic chemicals in water. Children have a bigger problem than do adults.

Rita Meyninger, president of Environmental Systems Management and Design in New Jersey, and Christopher Marlowe, a certified industrial hygienist, wrote about children at risk from water pollution in the May 1989 issue of *Civil Engineering.*[8]

They pointed out that the Clean Water Act may establish drinking-water standards based on the exposure of a healthy male adult who consumes eight cups of water per day. Infants and children, however, may be at greater risk than are adults from the same level of a toxic contaminant in a water supply. Because of their smaller size and their ability to absorb nutrients more efficiently than adults, Meyninger says, children have ten times the risk when they drink the same amount of polluted water as a healthy adult.*

Meyninger and Marlowe also point out that there are other exposure routes besides swallowing:

"Many light organic chemicals may be inhaled after they have been volatilized [made airborne] in showers, dishwashers, and washing machines, or they may be absorbed through the skin during bathing, showering, or swimming. This adds to the body burden of toxic chemicals in drinking water."

There are an estimated twelve thousand chemicals in water, and they can travel. So what an illegal dumper puts in the water six states away can end up in your glass. This was demonstrated by the National Water-quality Headquarters in the Robert A. Taft Sanitary Engineering Center in Cincinnati, Ohio. One day a water sample from St. Louis produced a peculiar new mark on a routine infrared test procedure. A week later, the same mark appeared in a test made from water sent in from New Orleans. The chemical had traveled hundreds of miles in the Mississippi River without undergoing any change, and showed up in one liter of water taken from the billions of gallons of water that pass through New Orleans every day.[9]

---

*For example, if a child weighing ten kilograms and an adult weighing seventy kilograms each drink two liters of water a day containing 3.5 milligrams per liter of a chemical, the child will receive a dosage three and half times that of the adult's.

In addition, children's gastrointestinal tracts are much more open to the passage of nutrients than are those of adults, and they absorb toxic agents more efficiently. If an adult absorbs 10 percent of a chemical administered orally and a child absorbs 30 percent, the child has triple the risk. With the two liters of water in the example above, the child's risk is ten times greater.

Industrial waste includes all manufacturing or other commercial waste that finds its way into water. The major contaminants are synthetic organic chemicals—solvents, cleansers, pesticides, fertilizers, gasoline additives, and other industrial, agricultural, and household products such as trihalomethanes and ethylene dichloride. Many of these synthetic organic chemicals do not break down into harmless components when they enter the environment. They may persist for many years. A number of them remain in water even after it is treated to kill bacteria and viruses; for chlorination, filtration, and other common water purification methods cannot—indeed are not intended to—remove synthetic organic chemicals.

As indicated by the incidents of industrial organic chemicals found in drinking water in Woburn and elsewhere, the result may be cancer, birth defects, or gene mutations.

While our municipal water systems have been assuring us that our water is perfectly safe, they really cannot be sure. Scientists are just now developing tests to try to detect some of these common, potentially harmful, organic chemicals in water.

TERRIBLE TIN

As this book is being written, several scientific conferences are being scheduled to discuss tin compounds, a newly recognized potentially harmful toxic pollutant in drinking water.

Tin compounds are rapidly increasing in use in industrial production as polyvinyl chloride stabilizers, catalysts, wood preservatives, marine antifouling agents, agricultural fungicides, insecticides, and moth and other insect repellents for use on fabrics.

Several preliminary investigations reveal that one tin compound, methyltin, may act like mercury, a known nerve toxin, in the environment. However, a method to detect minute amounts of tin substances in people or the environment has been lacking.

The widescale use of tin compounds was not seen as a problem in the past because early studies indicated that the substances would break down in water and sunlight to form harmless inorganic tin. The fact is that good tests to detect tin compounds in water were not available, so the complacency was not based on fact.

Methyltins constitute only a small portion of the tin compounds in industrial use. Dr. Michael Tompkins, now at Colorado State University in Fort Collins, reported in 1989 an analytical method that successfully measured about one part per billion of tin in a dozen samples of human urine. Eighteen percent of the tin in the urine samples was the toxic methyltins.

Commenting on the fact that the methyltin compounds displayed an increased solubility in fat-containing materials, the researchers said this points to the possible accumulation of these toxins in animal tissues and, concurrently, in the food chain.

Certain other tin compounds, trimethyltin and triethyltin, are known to be potent nerve toxins in mammals and are inhibitors of oxygen uptake in tissues and mitochondria, the powerhouses of the cell. The work of Dr. Frederick Brinckman and co-workers at the National Bureau of Standards showed that trimethyltin can transfer methyl groups (by "transmethylation") to mercury and other heavy metals to form highly toxic methylmercury and similar substances.

CADMIUM

Just as Dr. Braman was trying to work on methods to detect tin compounds in water, analytical chemist Ronald Smart at West Virginia University is trying to find accurate measurements of two other toxic metals, cadmium and lead, in natural waters. Dr. Smart says that even accurate measurements of the total amounts of those trace metals may not give a clear indication of the danger they pose.

"The trace metals we're studying are found in various forms, some evidently far more toxic than others. Yet currently used detection methods can't distinguish between the different forms," Dr. Smart said.

Most cadmium in natural waters comes from industrial discharges and mining waste. According to the Public Health Service, cadmium is a biologically nonessential, nonbeneficial element, and it is highly toxic. It can cause high blood pressure, abdominal cramps, kidney damage, difficulty with breathing and other symptoms.

Recognition of the serious toxic potential of cadmium when taken by mouth is based on reports of poisoning from cadmium-contaminated food and beverages, epidemiologic surveys that link cadmium with high blood pressure in humans under certain conditions, and long-term oral toxicity studies in animals, the Public Health Service said.

All levels of dietary cadmium, even as little as 0.1 mg per liter in drinking water, have caused cadmium accumulation in the soft tissues.

In a $100,000 research effort funded by the U.S. Environmental Protection Agency, Smart is developing techniques to measure only the more dangerous, free forms of cadmium and lead. He has designed an apparatus similar to a kidney dialysis machine, one that filters out trace metals bound up in large chemical complexes while it permits the free forms of cadmium and lead to pass through.

Smart plans to use his new technique to sample a wide range of water sources, from river water to acid mine drainage. This survey should begin to indicate what percentage of total cadmium and lead typically consists of the more toxic free metal. Smart says that in light of the new data federal guidelines may need to be reviewed and refined in terms of the free and total metal permitted.

LEAD

Lead is a more notorious and common pollutant than cadmium. The Environmental Protection Agency estimates that forty-two million Americans drink water that contains too much lead, more than 50 ppb of water. The EPA says that too much lead in the human body can cause serious damage to the brain, kidneys, nervous system, and red blood cells. It can cause fatigue and muscle soreness. The greatest risk, even with short-term exposure, is to young children and pregnant women.

In February 1989, small amounts of lead were found in the drinking water of three fountains in USA Today's news room on two floors of a modern office tower in Arlington, Virginia. Federal health experts investigated to determine whether the lead contamination could have been responsible for the fourteen miscarriages among eleven women on the news staff during the past year.

Excessive accumulation of lead in the body can cause severe learning disabilities and behavioral problems in children. In Scotland, 501 schoolchildren ages six to nine were tested for lead in their blood. Their mean blood lead level was 10.4 micrograms per dekaliter of blood, roughly half of what the United States Communicable Disease Centers consider "excessive." The Scots found that there was a 5.8 point differential in score results on the British Ability Scales between the least and most lead-exposed children. The British Ability Scales tests a child's ability to achieve in school. The higher the lead levels in students' blood, the lower their test scores.[10]

A similar report, of children in Boston filed in the *New England Journal of Medicine,* said that exposure to very low levels of lead before birth appears to slow children's mental development in their first years of life. *The study found dangers from lead even at levels thought to be safe for children.*

The children in the Boston lead study were not considered to be retarded, but their mental growth was slower than expected by the age of two.

The federal Centers for Disease Control considers lead levels to be unacceptable for children if they are higher than 25 micrograms in one millionth of a gram per deciliter of blood.[11]

On April 11, 1989, The EPA said that more than a million school water fountains still have lead components or lead-lined tanks, posing possible health risks to youngsters.[12]

The EPA considers a lead level of 20 ppb in water to pose health risks, especially if a child is exposed to lead from other sources as well. The agency estimates that lead in drinking water typically accounts for about 20 percent of the total exposure in young children.

What to Do About Lead

Manufacturing, mining, and coal burning are common sources of lead, and much of the lead from gasoline eventually enters natural water systems. Chances are, however, if you have lead in your water, it is not from a municipal reservoir but from old lead pipes that lead to your home or are in it, says Jack Winter, a water specialist affiliated with Jayson Water Systems in New Jersey.[13] He advises:

- If your home was built before the 1920s, it probably has water pipes made of lead; some of this lead will leach into water as it flows through the pipes.
- If your home was built between 1920 and 1950, your water pipes are probably made of iron, which is fine.
- If your home was built after 1950, lead solder may have been used to join copper piping. (Lead solder was banned in 1986.)

How can you tell whether your household pipes may be leaching lead into your water? Lead pipes are a dull gray color and are easily scratched with a knife or key. (The same is true of lead solder.)

Although hard water, Jack Winter says, may tend to coat the insides of your pipes, that coating helps protect your drinking water from any lead there may be in your water. On the other hand, if your water is soft or acidic, it can leach lead from the pipes.

How can you tell if you have soft water? You have it if it leaves a greenish spot in the sink and if the detergents and soaps you use really make a lot of suds. If you have installed your own water softener, consider disconnecting it from taps you use for drinking water.

Use a countertop charcoal water filter only if your lead problem isn't serious and you're diligent about changing the filter—about every four or five days. Left in place too long, a charcoal filter becomes a breeding ground for bacteria.

"If your plumbing contains lead, you should refrain from consuming water or cooking with water that sits in the pipes for several hours," Winter says. "Don't, for example, drink water from the tap the first thing in the morning or after you have returned from vacation. Flush your plumbing system by running the water for two to three minutes. Instead of running the water to waste, fill a few containers with water after the faucet has been used for some nonconsumptive use—for example, washing dishes or hands.

"Never use hot water for consumption or cooking— especially not for preparing baby formula. Hot water dissolves lead more quickly than does cold."

The WaterTest Corporation (see p. 201 for address and telephone number), which tests water in schools for lead, *has offered to test the water of readers of this book for $9.95* (regular cost, $30.95). Just send them a note mentioning the book's name.

The EPA says that since lead accumulates in your body, there is no safe level for lead in drinking water. However, if tests show that the level of lead in your water is 20 ppb or higher, you should reduce it immediately.

Winter says that if you do have lead in your drinking water, you should have the source—probably your household plumbing—changed. If you cannot have the pipes changed, or the source is from your water supply, then you can install a filtering system.

ALUMINUM

Drinking water with aluminum can increase the risk of contracting Alzheimer's disease by up to 50 percent, according to a publicly funded study published in the *Lancet,* the prestigious British medical journal.[14] The study was conducted by the Medical Research Council's epidemiology unit. People under seventy living in areas where the concentration of the mineral in drinking water is higher than 0.11 milligrams per liter had a 50 percent greater chance of contracting the disease, the study showed. The council examined levels of aluminum in drinking water over the past ten years in eighty-eight districts in England and Wales.

It was been widely reported that aluminum is found in the tangle of nerves and debris in the brains of Alzheimer's patients. However, many researchers believe that the aluminum is a result of the disease and not the cause. No one knows the answer for sure, as of this writing.

CHLORINE

A National Cancer Institute study, conducted in collaboration with investigators from research centers and health departments located around the country, suggests that people who have been drinking chlorinated surface water for forty or more years have an increased risk of developing bladder cancer.[15]

"The findings do not prove that this type of water causes bladder cancer, and they need to be confirmed in other studies," said chief investigator Dr. Kenneth Cantor of NCI's Environmental Epidemiology Branch. "Chlorinated drinking water offers immense health benefits, killing microorganisms that cause diseases like typhoid, cholera, polio, and hepatitis. The findings do not mean that we should stop disinfecting our water or drinking it."

Since chlorination began, waterborne disease has dropped dramatically in the United States. In contrast, the World Health Organization estimated that twenty-five thousand people die *each day* in the Third World from drinking contaminated or inadequately sanitized water.

"It is important to emphasize that cigarette smoking and occupational exposures are the chief causes of bladder cancer," Dr. Cantor said. About 70 percent of all bladder cancers among men and about 40 percent among women in the United States are due to smoking and occupational exposure. This year, an estimated 33,000 men and 12,400 women in the United States will be diagnosed with bladder cancer.

Approximately three-quarters of the U.S. population drinks chlorinated water, according to the Environmental Protection Agency's Office of Drinking Water. Although this estimate does not separate surface water (mainly from rivers, streams, and reservoirs) and groundwater (mainly from wells and springs), most chlorinated water is from surface water sources. Almost all large water systems are disinfected, and approximately half of the smaller groundwater systems are disinfected.

When chlorine is added to disinfect water, chlorination byproducts are formed, resulting from the interaction of chlorine with naturally occurring and man-made organic chemicals in the water. Surface waters usually have higher levels of these chemicals than does groundwater. Researchers have been concerned that some of the byproducts may increase cancer risk.

The NCI researchers found that risk for bladder cancer was affected by the combined influence of years of drinking chlorinated surface water and the amount consumed. Those who drank the largest amounts of this type of water daily (eight cups or more a day) for forty to fifty-nine years had a 40 percent increased risk compared with those who drank the least amounts (less than three and a half cups a day) and whose drinking water usually came from a non-chlorinated ground source. Those who drank the largest amounts of chlorinated surface water for forty years or more had an 80 percent increased risk.

The population-based, case-control study included data on white men and women, age twenty-one to eighty-four, about whom information was available regarding the type of drinking water they had consumed for at least half of their lives. Drinking water included tap water, as well as coffee, tea, and other beverages made with tap water.

Data were analyzed from 1,630 patients diagnosed with bladder cancer during the one-year period beginning December 1977, and from 3,027 individuals who did not have bladder cancer. The two groups were matched by age, sex, and geographic area.

It is not clear what compounds in the chlorinated surface water are responsible for the increased bladder cancer risk. Chlorination byproducts consist of volatile compounds, which evaporate upon heating, and nonvolatile compounds, which are not removed upon heating. "It is possible, however, that other contaminants in chlorinated surface water may be responsible for the increased risk," Dr. Cantor said.

If researchers find that certain byproducts are involved, it may be necessary to find ways to lower the levels of organic compounds that react with the chlorine or to explore other possible means of disinfecting drinking water.

Previous studies have suggested that chlorinated surface water is a risk factor for developing bladder cancer. These studies, however, were based on data from death certificates, while this new study was based on detailed information obtained directly from patient interviews. More case-control interview studies like this one will be needed to confirm the findings.

Ten geographic areas were included in the study: Atlanta, Detroit, New Orleans, San Francisco, Seattle, Connecticut, Iowa, New Jersey, New Mexico, and Utah. Detailed analyses of data by area were not possible in most cases because of limitations in data collection. In some areas, for example, there was not enough variation in the source of drinking water to allow comparison of groups by type of water. In some instances, the number of bladder cancer cases was too small, or there were not enough people for whom sufficient information was available on lifetime histories of drinking-water source.

The NCI study was supported in part by the Food and Drug Administration and the Environmental Protection Agency.

Fluorine, a relative of chlorine—both are halogenated nonmetallic elements—has been added in various forms to public water supplies to reduce the incidence of dental cavities. The concentration used has been purported to be far below the permissible level of toxicity of fluorine-containing compounds in the human body. The raw data from a federal study released by the National Toxicology Program (NTP) in January 1990 showed that rats fed fluoridated water developed two types of cancer: osteosarcoma, a bone cell cancer, and squamous carcinoma of the oral cavity.[16]

Upon release of the preliminary data, many anti-fluoridation activists said, "I told you so," while proponents of fluoridation said the amounts fed to the rats were much higher than those in public drinking water.

There is bound to be continuing debate about fluoridation as the NTP study progresses.

OTHER INDUSTRIAL POLLUTANTS

Besides tin, cadmium, aluminum, chlorine, and lead, there are many other elements that occur naturally in water or that are pollutants from industry. Here are physical problems caused by some of these pollutants in water:

- Copper causes anemia and heart disease. Water can be a significant source of copper intake, depending on where you live, the character of the water, the temperature of the water, and the presence of copper pipes. At concentrations about 1 mg per liter water, copper can stain laundry and plumbing fixtures. The presence of copper may also cause blonds to acquire a greenish-blue tint to their hair. Copper has toxic effects at high dosage levels and is an essential element at lower levels. Copper exposure at high levels may result in gastrointestinal disturbances and other acute toxic effects. Current maximum contaminated levels are 1 milligram per liter of water.

• Mercury causes manic depression and brain damage (see chapter 5).

• Volatile Organic Chemicals (VOCs) are synthetic compounds which readily become gases. Benzene is an example used in motor fuels, as a solvent, and in the manufacture of medicinal chemicals, dyes, and many other organic compounds. It is a human carcinogen.

WATER POLLUTION BY RUNOFF

In addition to industrial wastes in our waters, there is "natural pollution"—the leaching action of runoff water on natural deposits, forest soil, animal wastes, and chemically treated farmland.[17]

In the past fifty years, more than half a million new chemical compounds have come into existence. Many of them are discharged into our rivers and streams or dumped on the ground to seep into our underground water supplies.

Fish are good indicators of the dangers of polluted waters. Billions of fish have died in the past twenty-five years from chemicals in our streams, rivers, lakes, and oceans. Amazingly small amounts of pesticides can kill shrimp, crab, and other aquatic life. One part DDT in a billion parts of water was found to kill blue crabs in eight days. The relationship is the same as one ounce of chocolate syrup to ten million gallons of milk.[18] The warning is clear. What is bad for the fish is bad for humans.

What chemical is the principal "natural" water pollutant? Nitrogen, mostly in nitrates. Water gets it both from urban and industrial waste and from agricultural fertilizers.

A landmark article on well water and methemoglobinemia (lack of oxygen in the blood) in infants, caused by nitrates in well water, was written by a pediatric resident, Hunter Comly, M.D., who sought to discover the cause of cyanosis (a dark blue color of the skin due to lack of oxygen in the blood) in two infants in Iowa[19]. One father suspected that his child's recurrent cases of blue skin and difficulty in breathing were caused by well water. Dr. Comly had the water from the suspect well analyzed and demonstrated that well-water nitrates can cause methemoglobinemia in infants. A survey of wells in Iowa then clearly demonstrated the public health dimension of the problem.

The contributions of Comly's case reports are several. The most important is the recognition of nitrates as the cause of methemoglobinemia in infants who were fed milk formulas reconstituted or diluted with contaminated well water. The likely magnitude of the problem was assessed by soliciting information about similar cases from other physicians and by measuring the nitrate content of water obtained from ninety-one Iowa wells. More than 50 percent of the water samples contained nitrate nitrogen in excess of 10 ppm (parts per million), the level permitted by the Environmental Protection Agency, and 20 percent contained more than 65 ppm. An article in the *Journal of the American Medical Association* in 1987 said that despite public health surveillance and physician education, toxic methemoglobinemia remains a potentially lethal problem for infants in rural America. The article noted that in a 1981 survey of a thousand wells in South Dakota, 27 percent were contaminated by nitrates in concentrations that exceed the EPA's permissible limit.[20]

Runoff from agricultural products (such as nitrates) and from industrial wastes overfertilize aquatic plant life and result in the process known as eutrophication. When water supplies are taken from lakes or streams that are undergoing eutrophication, the algae affect treatment plant operations, cause clogging of filters, may cause undesirable tastes and odor, and impair water quality.

Just as scientists have found that individually harmless chemicals, when combined in food or drugs, may become toxic, they have also found the same thing in water. Water chemists refer to such combinations as "gunk." For example, two parts per million copper won't hurt fish, nor eight parts zinc. But *combine* one-tenth of these amounts and all the fish in the streams will die.

GETTING IN HOT WATER

In addition to industrial waste and runoff water pollution, there is *thermal pollution*—the addition of hot waters from nuclear plants and other industries that upsets the oxygen balance, opening the door to other pollutants.

WATERBORNE DISEASE

Illness from unseen industrial pollutants may take years to develop, but often diseases from sewage pollution, from raw or partly treated domestic waste, can occur quite rapidly after ingestion.

In mid-January 1987, a college physician informed health authorities of a dramatic increase in gastroenteritis among students at West Georgia College in Carrollton, Georgia. The hospital reported that the telltale parasite eggs of cryptosporidium were found in the stool of four patients. Cryptosporidium causes sudden, severe diarrhea and abdominal cramps. Stools of patients with cryptosporidiosis are highly infectious and there is no uniformly effective therapy available. The disease is usually self-limiting except in patients whose immune systems are compromised; then it can be fatal.[21]

An investigation showed that between January 12 and February 7, 1987, an outbreak of intestinal upsets affected an estimated 13,000 people in a county of 64,900 residents.[22] The sudden onset of widespread gastroenteritis affecting persons of all ages is typical of a waterborne outbreak.

Cryptosporidium eggs were identified in the stools of 58 of 147 patients with gastroenteritis tested during the outbreak. Cryptosporidium eggs were also identified in samples of treated public water with use of monoclonal antibodies (high-tech tests that only recently have become available). Although the sand-filtered and chlorinated water system met all regulatory-agency quality standards, inadequate filtration probably allowed the parasite to pass into the drinking-water supply. Low-level cryptosporidium infection in cattle in the watershed and a sewage overflow were considered as possible contributors to the contamination of the surface water supply. This became the first reported contamination of a filtered water system by cryptosporidium. The Center for Disease Control researchers subsequently concluded that current standards for the treatment of public water supplies may not prevent the contamination of drinking water by cryptosporidium, with consequent outbreaks of cryptosporidiosis.

Contamination of rivers and streams by cryptosporidium has been reported in several states, and the investigation shows that it can contaminate filtered public water systems—even when the water quality is within regulatory limits for coliform bacteria, chlorine, and turbidity—causing large epidemics of gastroenteritis in otherwise healthy persons.

GIARDIA

Cryptosporidium eggs are a newly recognized water problem and so is *Giardia lamblia,* a protozoan that is a danger in drinking water.

In the 1980s, thousands of people in Missoula, Montana, and hundreds of others in northeastern Pennsylvania and Vermont were made ill by drinking their municipal water from taps in their homes. The culprit was a microscopic parasite, *Giardia lamblia,* which causes severe diarrhea.[23]

A generation ago, the *Giardia* parasite was believed to dwell amicably in the human digestive tract. Then, in 1966, *Giardia* was identified as the cause of an outbreak of intestinal disease in Aspen, Colorado, after the water supply became contaminated with sewage. *Giardia* contamination is now recognized as a worldwide problem, and it is believed that 2 to 10 percent of the population carries the parasite in their intestines.

Giardia is one reason you should not drink water from even a pristine-appearing stream since it is often swimming invisibly in the water. What is even more worrisome, *Giardia* can also swim in chlorinated municipal water.[24]

VIRUSES

In the first edition of *Poisons in Your Food,* Dr. Luther L. Terry, surgeon general of the Public Health Service in 1961, said: "When I entered the Public Health Service some twenty years ago, I was taught by the senior physicians of our Corps that whatever else in our environment was dangerous to health, our water supplies were safe. But three dangers are causing us to re-examine our water's spotless reputation."[25] Dr. Terry listed virus diseases, new chemicals, and radiation. Radiation has not been found to be a major problem, but certainly chemicals and viruses have been.

Virus diseases are borne in human feces. Water inspectors determine the level of contamination of our drinking water by measuring *Escherichia coli,* which is present in fecal matter from humans and other mammals. Its presence is an indication of contamination (see pages 170–172).

Two families of viruses are excreted from the feces: the enteroviruses—which include polio, Coxsackie, and Echo viruses—and the adenoviruses. The enteroviruses multiply in the human intestines and are discharged in the feces. Adenoviruses apparently multiply in the human intestines, too, and are also found in the feces, but less is known about them. Adenoviruses are associated with upper respiratory diseases causing inflammation of the mucous membrane of the respiratory system and of the eyes.

EPA FILE REVELATIONS

The National Wildlife Federation study "Danger on Tap" reviewed EPA files and found that more than 110,000 people became ill from drinking contaminated water from 1971 to 1985, more people than in any other previous fourteen-year period.

That number may be underestimated as much as twenty-five times because it only includes people who became ill immediately after drinking contaminated water and fails to take into account long-term illnesses like cancer that may be caused by polluted water.[26]

According to an audit conducted by the EPA's inspector general in September 1988, not only had the agency ignored 100,000 violations of federal standards by public water systems, it also was not enforcing regulations governing 150,000 noncommunity water systems used by about thirty-six million people in restaurants, schools, motels, and industries that have their own wells or reservoirs.

The audit said the agency's failure to monitor compliance with water standards aboard airlines, trains, and buses resulted in "passengers traveling on these interstate carrier conveyances . . . being exposed to unnecessary health risks."

The Safe Drinking Water Act of 1974—passed five years after the first edition of *Poisons in Your Food* was published—applied the first National Interim Primary Drinking Water regulations to all public water supplies in the United States. The Act was stimulated by a 1970 study that showed that approximately eight million Americans were drinking potentially harmful water from approximately five thousand public water supplies. The EPA was delegated to oversee the development and enforcement of regulations. Standards were set for one microbial agent (coliform bacteria), ten inorganic chemicals, six pesticides, and radionuclides.

The 1986 amendments to the Safe Drinking Water Act called for the immediate regulation of eighty-three contaminants, followed by regulation of twenty-five more at designated intervals. Among the microbial agents named were *Legionella,* the causative agent of legionnaire's disease, which was identified in 1976; *Giardia,* the chief pathogen associated with waterborne disease in the United States; and viruses long associated with waterborne outbreaks of disease.

The chemical contaminants fell into several categories: those that occur naturally, such as radon (which causes lung cancer) and arsenic (which causes skin cancer); those that are man-made, such as pesticides and organic solvents (pesticides and PCBs attack the central nervous system and cause depression and irrational behavior); and those that derive from the materials used in supplying water, most notably asbestos and lead. The act specifically banned the use of lead pipes, solder, and flux in the installation or repair of any public water system and called for the regulation of disinfectants and their byproducts in water.

Cryptosporidium—described above—is not among the eighty-three regulated contaminants because it is a newly recognized human pathogen. Cryptosporidium does appear on the list of contaminants scheduled for regulation in 1991, but its regulation will depend on whether adequate treatments are available.

Congress may have passed the legislation, but it failed to provide adequate funding. The EPA abolished its section on the health effects of microbial agents and transferred these responsibilities to the monitoring section. Little research is being done on the relative health risk posed by parasites, viruses, and bacteria in potable water to the more than thirty million Americans who have reduced immune function, according to Betty H. Olson, Ph.D., of the University of California, in an editorial in the *New England Journal of Medicine*:

"The chemical contaminant picture is no brighter. Although relatively more money is spent in this area to develop risk-assessment data, the list of possibly hazardous chemicals in water grows ever longer. . . . Given its heavy responsibility for protecting the public, it is hard to believe that research is not a legislated part of the EPA's mission."[27]

In 1987 the EPA was unable to enforce water-safety standards for lack of money. It neglected to act on more than a hundred thousand violations in water systems serving thirty-seven million people. And an audit in September 1988 found that the agency was not enforcing water-quality regulations for airlines, trains, and buses.

The Environmental Protection Agency on June 22, 1989, adopted stricter rules to try to eliminate harmful germs from the nation's public drinking water, preventing some ninety thousand cases of waterborne disease a year.[28]

The rules, mandated by Congress when it amended the Clean Water Act in 1986, may require many systems that rely on surface water, including New York City's, to install expensive filtration systems. EPA officials noted that it will cost three billion dollars in capital costs and five hundred million dollars a year for operation and maintenance of pollution control equipment. The systems would be used to destroy bacteria, viruses, protozoa, and other waterborne organisms that cause diseases like hepatitis A, giardiasis, and legionnaire's disease.

In compliance, the agency announced standards for dealing with six specific waterborne organisms, required many water systems to install filtration equipment, and increased the monitoring of drinking water. Under the rules, state governments will determine whether filtration must be installed to meet the federal standards.

Until 1989, the agency had set no specific standards for limiting water contamination for most of the organisms. Water utilities relied chiefly on chlorine and other disinfectants. "We have made remarkable progress in protecting public health from waterborne disease," said William K. Reilly, administrator of the EPA. But he added, "We still see many illnesses resulting from poor treatment at the supply plant or contamination problems in the distribution systems."[29]

Water utility managers welcomed the rules. John H. Sullivan, deputy executive director for governmental affairs of the American Water Works Association, a professional group that represents the utilities, said the association has been advocating filtration of surface water supplies for some years.

However, the rules do not apply to underground water.

The EPA estimated that under its new rule, fifteen hundred public water systems that rely on surface water would have to install filtration, five thousand systems would have to improve their existing filtration, and another thirty-five hundred systems would have to improve their disinfection programs or find other sources of water.

In addition, all two hundred thousand water supply systems in the United States that serve twenty-five or more people, whether they use surface or underground water, will have to improve monitoring for coliforms, bacteria that are generally not harmful themselves but are an indication of potentially dangerous fecal wastes in water.

WHAT YOU CAN DO

- *Take a simple water test.* This can help you determine the presence of detergents or other organic materials present in a river, well, or glass of water. This particular test was devised by George J. Crits, assistant technical manager of the Cochrane Division of the Crane Company, Philadelphia. Take a tall, cylindrical bottle such as a baby bottle or one in which olives are packed. Fill it half full of water, stopper it, and shake it. The presence of high amounts of detergents or soap will cause a noticeable foam. Small amounts will cause a film that will travel upward on the side of the glass bottle. The film rises until it disappears at a height that depends on the amount of contamination in the water. The greater that contamination, the greater the height of the film or ring.

- *Hold a public hearing.* The Safe Drinking Water Act empowers any citizen to petition the EPA to hold a public hearing to bring a water utility into compliance with the law. When all else fails, you can sue a water system, the state, or the EPA to compel compliance.

- *Organize and sue.* A New Jersey electroplating company, Arrow Group Industries, Inc., kept dumping zinc and chromium into a brook trout stream. A New Jersey public interest research group and Friends of the Earth brought a suit against Arrow and won a $600,000 settlement. The money was used to help improve the ability to handle toxic heavy metals in the rivers and other aquatic environment.[30]

- *If you have a private well, have it tested.* According to nationwide estimates, between 15 and 20 percent of all private wells in the United States have levels of volatile chemicals above the legislative mandate. Your state Environmental Protection Agency should have a list of certified water-test companies. WaterTest Corporation, mentioned on page 189, (address below), will perform home testing, as will Watercheck, 6151 Wilson Mills Road, Cleveland, Ohio 44143 (800-458-3330). Some water experts suggest private wells be checked annually, at least for bacteria and nitrates, and once every three years for total dissolved solids and pH (acidity) levels.

- *Check for lead in your household water supply.* You can contact WaterTest Corporation, Box 6360, Manchester, New Hampshire 03108-6360 (800-426-8378), which offers a special rate of $9.95 for readers of this book (just mention the title) or you can order House-Chek, a home test for lead, for twenty dollars from Diagnostics and Devices, Inc., 1201 Mount Kemble Avenue, Morristown, New Jersey 07960.

- *If you need a home water-filtering system, check carefully before you buy.* There are many home-treatment devices, ranging in price from twenty-five dollars for a faucet filter to over a thousand dollars for a total in-house treatment plant. State health officials warn that faucet filters can build up bacteria and various other substances if they are not properly maintained. The EPA does not certify or approve home water filters, but it does make information available on tests performed on the filters. For details, write EPA Public Inquiries Center (PM-215), 401 M Street S.W., Washington, D.C. 20460.

- *If you are on a low-salt or salt-free diet, be aware that water softeners add as much as 351 mg of sodium per liter of water.* The level of 20 mg of sodium/liter of drinking water is suggested by the EPA for the population at high risk for high blood pressure and/or heart disease.
- *Buy bottled water.* This is a simple but more expensive way to solve the problem. Again, make sure the bottled water you are buying is pure. There is a controversy over bottled water versus tap water. Some say the municipal water is often purer, and in some cases it *is* the water in the bottle. Do some library research for current evaluations by *Consumer Reports* and other organizations, and check with the Bottled Water Association, 113 N. Henry Street, Alexandria, Virginia 22314.

Below are some terms that will help you understand the different kinds of water available:

- Municipal water: may contain chlorine, fluorine.
- Spring water: comes from the underground to surface naturally; contains minerals.
- Mountain spring water: same as spring water except remoteness of spring may ensure it is uncontaminated.
- Purified water: tap or underground water that is rendered mineral-free.
- Sparkling water: carbon dioxide may be present (naturally sparkling) or may be added.
- Seltzer water: usually municipal water that has been filtered and carbonated.
- Club soda: same as seltzer, with minerals and mineral salts added.

8 ⌐ Eating Out Tonight?

As I stood in line at a barbecue in an exclusive tennis and swim club whose members are among the most intelligent and well-to-do in New Jersey, the French chef behind the table, cigarette dangling from his mouth, was dishing out spaghetti with his fingers. He was sweating profusely. An elderly gentleman in front of me complained loudly at such an obvious breach of sanitation and stalked out of the club. I stayed, fascinated by a flagrant violation of the most elementary health practices involved in serving food to the public.

Farther down the line, I saw a young assistant spooning desserts on a plate and stopping every once in a while to lick his fingers. The waitresses, hired for the summer, had long hairdos that hung loose over the food they served. Flies were plentiful. I looked at the silverware; some of it was encrusted with food. A meat sandwich that was served had obviously been sliced from meat that had been cooked the day before, for it was dry and unappetizing.

I was reminded of what I had learned from food inspectors: much of what I saw actually goes on in many of the more than half a million eating places in the United States. The difficulty is that the patrons just don't see it, for most of it takes place behind the scenes, in the kitchens and larders.

One young chef told me recently how she quit an "in" restaurant on the New Jersey coast without giving notice.

"The owners were defrosting a turkey on the counter," she said. "The kitchen wasn't even air-conditioned. The help was sweating. When I objected to defrosting the turkey that way, the owners said that's the way they do it and that was the way it was going to be done. I took off my apron and left!"

We Americans spend 42.1 percent of our food dollars away from home. We buy twenty-eight billion meals a year at 720,000 food service places, spending $179.7 billion dollars. We are eating an increasingly large proportion of our meals at fast-food restaurants. When this book was first published, sales at "limited menu" places accounted for about 14 percent of the total food service industry. Today, fast-food restaurants are 28.2 percent of total food service and account for 43.5 percent of all sales in public eating places.[1]

Routine inspection of restaurants to prevent foodborne disease is mandated by food sanitation codes throughout the United States. But the shrinking tax dollar together with mounting public pressures for prevention of environmental pollution have placed food protection programs in fierce competition with other environmental programs such as air, water, and solid-waste programs. Not only are community health inspectors required to investigate restaurants, they also investigate dog bites, ragweed pollution, swimming pools, sewage, garbage, pet shops, gasoline stations, citizens' complaints, rodents, smoke, and other nuisances.

Charles W. Felix, M.P.H., of Charles Felix Associates, Leesburg, Virginia, and publisher of *Food Protection Report*, said there was a time when a restaurant was subject to twelve health department inspections a year. Nowadays, the health inspector may get to a restaurant once in twelve months. In the meantime, there are eight million pairs of hands involved in serving food to the public, two million of them teenaged hands. (When was the last time your teenager washed his hands?) With that many hands in the pot, it is inevitable that some o. the broth will be spoiled and some of us will fall ill. It's the nature of the game.[2]

"Have you ever been ill from a foodborne disease?" Felix asked. "I have been on a number of occasions when I was never quite sure whether it was from 'something I ate' or from 'something that was going around.' But on one occasion, I was involved in an outbreak in which dozens of people fell ill from something we all ate at a buffet—the social opening, by the way, of a public health convention, the annual educational conference of the Environmental Health Association in Las Vegas, Nevada, in 1970. While I was made very uncomfortable for a day, there were a number of the conventioneers who were hospitalized with severe gastrointestinal disorders."

Thirty-two percent of foodborne illnesses reported to the Centers for Disease Control began in the kitchens of commercial eating places.[3]

The National Restaurant Association (NRA) notes that out of a total of 45 billion meals eaten in restaurants, schools, and work cafeterias each year, the annual incidence of foodborne disease attributable to food service establishments is only about one in every 160,000 meals. Of course, if you or a loved one is *that one,* you really are upset. Furthermore, many people do not associate an illness with the food eaten hours and even days earlier at a restaurant, and if they do, they frequently take no action.

What causes such outbreaks, the restaurant personnel?

In the first edition of *Poisons in Your Food,* Dr. Aaron Haskins, health officer for Newark, New Jersey, explained that in 1921, the city of Newark passed an ordinance requiring the physical examination of food handlers, the theory being that a sick food handler would transmit disease through food. Dr. Haskins said,

> While the theory is commendable, the actual practice cannot be considered so. The physical examination consisted of an X ray of the chest, blood serology, and a mouth smear. The examination also included a very cursory screening for superficial skin infections. If we realize that the diseases most apt to spread through food are of the salmonella, typhoid and dysentery groups staphylococcus and streptococcus organisms, you can readily see that the type of examination as carried out is not directed at these organisms; the program has degenerated into a case-finding program for tuberculosis and venereal disease.
>
> The fallacy of the physical examination for the prevention of the spread of disease through food becomes more obvious when we realize that even if we were able to carry out the

proper type of examination, it would only show that at the time of examination the food handler was well. But the next day he could easily become infected with any of these important diseases, and be a source of infection, and still have in his possession a health card from a health department testifying that he is well and that it is safe for him to handle food.

In my opinion, this gives the public and the food handler a false sense of security, because unless that food handler is acquainted with the disease that he may have and unless he knows how to properly conduct himself so that he may not infect the food, the public is not safe. I believe that no physical examination of the food handler is the answer to this problem and certainly the public should not be lulled into this false sense of security.[4]

Many food handlers in American restaurants today are immigrants from countries where they worried more about obtaining enough to eat than about hygiene. Furthermore, many of them have parasites that can and are being transmitted to the food they handle. As Dr. Haskins pointed out twenty years ago, experience has shown that even if you do rid the food handlers of their worms and other parasites, they soon become reinfected by members of their own households.

What about food handlers and AIDS, that devastating, immunity-destroying disease that was not even considered when the first edition of this book was published?

The NRA does not consider AIDS a threat if a food handler is a victim of the disease. The NRA publication *Make a S.A.F.E. Choice: A Sanitary Assessment of Food Environment: A New Approach to Restaurant Self-Inspection* states: "Let's make it abundantly clear: the virus which causes AIDS is *not* spread by food. The U.S. Public Health Service, Centers for Disease Control says, 'Because AIDS is not transmitted through preparation or serving of food and beverages . . . food service workers infected with AIDS should not be restricted from work unless they have another infection or illness for which such restrictions would be warranted.' "[5]

More than twenty years ago, Dr. Haskins identified the answer to much of the problem of food safety in restaurants, and today almost everyone agrees that it lies in educating food handlers about sanitation. Since kitchen help are often paid very little when compared with other occupations, many employees suffer from lack of formal education and may not be aware of the need for sanitary handling of food.

Education of food handlers is difficult to implement. The turnover of restaurant help is almost 100 percent each year.

Since the early 1970s, the United States Food and Drug Administration has worked on guidelines for the improved dissemination of information and training about food protection and sanitation in food-service establishments, food stores, and the food-vending industry. The agency has worked with local state health departments to establish training programs for managers and to develop tests to determine if the information is being understood and retained.

How many people does the FDA have available to work with state health departments, restaurant inspectors, supermarkets, and other food-service places? Five—four inspectors and one administrator.

Still, cooperation among federal, state, county, and city health officials as well as the food-service industry has led to a substantial improvement in education of food handlers.

The National Restaurant Association, which says there are 270,698 restaurants in the nation, has made great efforts to help members educate employees about sanitation. *Make a S.A.F.E. Choice* stresses that the cost to restaurants can be very high when customers are made ill because of mishandling of food. The following examples were given:

- The caterer didn't refrigerate the roast beef; 112 customers became ill with *Clostridium perfringens*. The direct cost to the restaurant, $21,218.
- The kitchen staff left the egg batter out overnight; 119 customers were infected with *Salmonella* and 50 percent of the staff was laid off for six weeks, until they could prove they had negative stool samples. The direct cost to the restaurant, $89,000.

- The manager decided to use home-canned peppers; 53 people were hospitalized with botulism and the restaurant closed for five months. The direct cost to the restaurant, $571,000.
- The chef kept the béarnaise sauce at room temperature; 26 customers developed *Staphylococcus* intoxication; one victim suffered total paralysis, and the restaurant was closed permanently. Direct cost to the restaurant, $1,051,600.[6]

The National Restaurant Association says that the average cost to implicated restaurants in an outbreak of foodborne diseases is $73,858 in medical charges, lost wages, lost business, lawyers' fees, and legal claims. Since ill customers are likely to sue the restaurant for damages, this leads to increases in liability insurance premiums.

Every restaurant, therefore, has a great stake in keeping its customers not only happy but healthy.

In advising its members on how to react if something does go wrong and people do complain about illness from a meal eaten in their restaurants, the NRA points out that members of the same family or dining party can often convince each other that they are ill. "But if several persons unrelated to each other all report the same illness and the same food experience, this increases the chances that the complaints are legitimate, and you should investigate it."[7] The NRA advises its members to:

- Get all the pertinent information possible.
- Remain polite and concerned, but don't argue and don't admit liability.
- Let the person tell his own story—don't introduce symptoms.
- Do not diagnose or advise on treatment.

The best protection against foodborne illness is education, as this book emphasizes over and over again. A food handler who knows proper methods of storing, preparing, and serving food protects the customer's health.

Educational Testing Services (ETS), Princeton, New Jersey, has developed a certification program that tests food handlers' knowledge of food hygiene.

Charles Felix pointed out that because the Educational Testing Food Protection Certification Program is independent of any one form of training, it encourages many different types of training programs, including home study courses, community college curricula, a video instructional program, and in-house industry programs—the food worker is free to select the medium of instruction he or she feels is most suitable.

Pat Silvers of Educational Testing Services said that 7,600 food handlers took the test in 1988 and 5,547 passed.[8] ETS does not itself provide any training but does offer a three-dollar booklet on preparing to take the test. Because ETS maintains a national registry of certified managers, these workers will be able to carry their certifications with them to other parts of the country.

The Public Health Service does have thick files on outbreaks of food poisoning, although personnel admit that their records are just the very tip of the iceberg. Such illnesses are not all from germs. Take the classic case of the barbecue-stand patron who loved chili. He ate some "mexihot." Six hours later, he was dead. On the same day, when several other patrons became ill, food sanitarians traced the case to a roadside stand. The chef refused to believe it, and ate some chili himself to prove his point. He died.[9] Though there were no disease germs in the food, the laboratory discovered a quantity of sodium fluoride, a poison used for killing roaches, in the chili.

In another incident, 236 people on the West Coast got sick because roach powder had been mistaken for powdered milk and mixed with some scrambled eggs. Forty-seven died.

Although the above incidents happened years ago, the Alameda County Health Care Services Agency investigators in California decided to explore the current routes of industrial chemicals in food served in restaurants. They investigated two hundred restaurants and found a number of health risks related to the use and storage of cleansers, food additives, and pesticides. Steven R. Anderson, Registered Sanitarian of the Alameda County Health Care Services Agency, said the Centers for Disease Control report for 1981 showed that approximately 20 percent of all foodborne outbreaks were caused by chemicals.[10] Among chemical poisoning outbreaks originating from food-service establishments in 1981 were monosodium glutamate, trisodium phosphate, sodium hydroxide, heavy metals, calcium chloride, and cleaning agents.

In two restaurants, Anderson said, caustic solutions were found to have leaked from grill-cleaning products. Thus it is important that cleansers not be stored directly above food preparation areas.

In one restaurant, which did not have professional pest control services, rodent bait in open trays was found on walk-in cooler shelves where foods were also stored. In another restaurant, an automatic device for dispensing pyrethrin and piperonyl butoxide was found mounted directly over exposed foods.

Anderson said that the FDA banned coumarin as a food additive more than thirty years ago because it was shown to cause cancer. Yet a survey and laboratory work performed in May 1984 revealed that 54 percent (seven out of thirteen samples) of Mexican vanilla available to Alameda County's residents contained coumarin.

In a March 1984 incident, a disinfectant, sodium hydroxide, was kept in a green wine bottle while the restaurant's dishwasher was broken. When the bottle was almost empty, it was inadvertently put back on the shelf and refilled with wine. The patron who was served a drink from that container suffered severe burning of the esophagus.

In another case, potatoes were soaked in a concentrated anti-oxidant solution of sulfites overnight rather than for one and a half minutes, as recommended on the label.

Anderson concluded that in Alameda County all Mexican vanilla was considered suspect and sellers were advised to remove the product. Automatic dispensing units containing pyrethrin were to be allowed providing the units were timed to release when the business was closed, and foods were at least twelve feet from the devices.

For the sake of the sulfite sensitive, efforts are being made to provide written warnings in restaurants where sulfiting agents are used (through posted signs or menu notices).

The Alameda researchers found that indiscriminate use of caustic cleansers can lead to direct contamination of foods; excessive use of preservatives during food preparation may result in chemical poisoning; and improper storage and use of pesticides in food establishments can result in food contamination or produce adverse effects in customers.[11]

The National Restaurant Association says that investigation of foodborne disease outbreaks consistently reveals that the major factors causing bacterial illnesses are:

1. Preparing foods several hours or more in advance of service.
2. Inadequate hot storage of foods.
3. Inadequate cooking of foods.
4. Inadequate reheating of foods.
5. Contamination of foods from infected workers or other sources.[12]

What do health inspectors look for routinely when evaluating a restaurant?

The inspectors ask

- Are the cold foods, including cream pies and custards, kept under proper refrigeration (below 45°F)?
- Are the hot foods not kept hot enough (steam tables should be 140°F)?
- Are foods stored properly? (If onions and flour are stored on the floor, for example, they are being stored improperly.)
- Are displayed foods protected by glass?
- Does food splash on single-service items such as paper cups?
- Are there open sugar bowls? Sugar should be served in individual packages or in a closed container.
- What are the toilet facilities like? Can the help wash their hands in a convenient place?
- Are there cross-connections with or back-siphonage into the water supply from sinks, dishwashing machines, lavatories, or toilets? There shouldn't be.
- Does the drain from the steam tables reflush over the tables (a common violation)?
- Are the grease traps in good repair, clean and unclogged?
- Are insect strips placed away from food or are they hung over tables used for preparation of food where condensation from the heat causes them to drip into the food and milk? (Fly leg in your

soup? To help prevent that from happening, the Food and Drug Administration asked the Agricultural Research Service to find out how far fly parts scatter when house flies are caught in electrocuting traps. To be safe, the USDA found, wall-mounted traps should be six feet away from food areas, while ceiling-hung traps should be ten feet away.)[13]

- Has food been left out overnight?
- Has garbage been covered and disposed of promptly?
- Have insect and rodent killers been kept far away from the food?
- Have dishes been washed either by hot water in a dishwashing machine or disinfected with chemicals?
- What is the source of the restaurant's food supplies?
- Is anyone smoking while food is being prepared?
- Do employees wear headbands, hairnets, or caps, and are all uniforms clean?[14]

All of these questions make sense, of course, but restaurant inspection itself is controversial. When Dr. George Kupchik, director of environmental health of the American Public Health Association, was asked by the author whether he felt confident when he went into a restaurant that was not inspected by a health department, he said, "I don't feel confident when I go into a restaurant that I know is inspected! Restaurants inspected every three months for ten years are no better than restaurants that have never been inspected," he said. "There is no question in my mind that some of the fanciest-name restaurants lack adequate sanitation. On the other hand, some small, family-run eating places have excellent sanitation."[15]

Seattle, Washington, health inspectors, however, showed recently that *restaurant inspection can pinpoint conditions that will lead to foodborne outbreaks.*

There are 3,076 restaurants in the Seattle–King County Department of Public Health's area. Sanitarians in five health districts use a standard reporting form developed by the Seattle–King County department of health. Data from the current form have been entered into a computerized inspection file since the form was adopted on January 1, 1986. The form identifies forty-two types of violations classified as "critical" or "noncritical." Critical violations—for example, the temperature of potentially hazardous foods, food-handling practices, the health status of food handlers—are thought to have direct impact on foodborne disease. Noncritical items, such as the cleanliness of nonfood contact surfaces, are thought to play a minor role in foodborne illnesses.

A score of less than 70 points indicates a "suspend permit."

Epidemiologists in the Seattle–King County Department of Public Health receive about seven hundred complaints of suspected foodborne illness each year. All suspected outbreaks are investigated. A reported outbreak of foodborne illness is defined as "an incident in which two or more persons have the same disease, have similar symptoms, or excrete the same germ after eating a common food or beverage."[16] Poisoning by botulism or by a toxic chemical requires only one ill individual to elicit investigation.

Although thirty-six restaurants were associated with an outbreak during the period of study, only twenty-eight were permanent facilities with an active permit and therefore eligible for further analyses. Controls were similar restaurants with no outbreaks.

The foodborne outbreaks affected from one to six persons. The implicated germ was unknown for most outbreaks; poultry was the most commonly implicated food. The implicated contributory cause for most outbreaks was improper temperature control of food during cooking, cooling, reheating, holding, or storage. The interval between inspection and outbreak ranged from 2 to 14.1 months, with a mean interval of 3.7 months. This interval is less than the four-month inspection interval recommended for all restaurants by the Seattle–King Country Public Health Department.

Restaurants with an overall score of less than 86 (out of 100) were about five times more likely to have a subsequent outbreak of food poisoning than were those with better scores. Restaurants that received an inspection result of "unsatisfactory" or "suspend permit" were about three times more likely to "poison" their customers than were those with satisfactory results.

Large restaurant size may represent a risk factor simply because such restaurants serve numerous patrons, thus increasing the likelihood of finding two ill persons needed to identify an outbreak, the Seattle inspectors said. Alternatively, large restaurants may be more likely to have an outbreak because of poor control of food temperatures, greater food volume, more complex menus, or less closely supervised food handlers. The association of the outbreaks with corporate ownership largely reflects the outbreaks with restaurant size.

The Seattle investigators said that it may be just chance that during inspections Chinese and other Asian restaurants were cited more than were other restaurants, but certain food preparation practices in Cantonese-style restaurants have been found to be hazardous.

American cuisine had a clearly negative association with outbreaks, the Seattle study concluded.

The Seattle health department functions are much admired by professional sanitarians around the country. In many other areas of the country, inspection of restaurants by civil employees is not even adequate. Half the people performing restaurant inspections in New York City, for example, were arrested in 1988 for extortion. In all, there are approximately forty to eighty people responsible for inspecting the city's fourteen thousand restaurants at least once a year and reinspecting those that fail their first checkup. But as health inspectors, they also have to inspect single-room occupancy hotels, dairies, camps, pools, and new restaurants for licensing. Among their other duties, they are responsible for checking out public complaints about restaurants, pollution, and vermin. Their pay? About $19,000 to $22,000 a year. Requirements? A bachelor's degree with thirty science credits.

To Samuel Leff, who wrote about his experience in "Corruption in the Kitchen," an article in the October 17, 1988, issue of *New York* magazine, the job of health inspector requires intelligence, skill, tact, and resourcefulness, and it is dangerous. He said he was attacked once and seriously threatened several times by angry restaurant owners.

"My work exposed me to many kinds of toxic fumes. For instance, when word passed through a kitchen that an inspector was out front, employees often frantically saturated infested areas with potent insect sprays clearly marked 'FOR USE BY LICENSED EXTERMINATORS ONLY.' "

Leff said he asked one of the staffers at the Health Academy where inspectors are trained why the salaries were so low for health inspectors.

"Bribes," Leff was told. "They're making enough from bribes so they don't need to push for better salaries."[17]

The person who is underpaid in a job like inspector is vulnerable to bribes.

Food inspectors may be absolutely honest and highly skilled at their jobs, but they too can make mistakes. The fallibility of inspection was demonstrated in an item from *FDA Papers*:

"Two Philadelphia FDA inspectors developed severe symptoms of food poisoning after eating at a diner in Allentown, Pa. One required hospital treatment. Investigation showed that the diner used drinking water from a contaminated well and stored and handled food in an unsanitary manner. Bacteriological findings in sausage and butter samples taken at the diner were reported to the State of Pennsylvania Department of Health."

You can criticize food handlers and restaurant bosses for improper handling of food, but what about the customers?

Salad bars were introduced in the 1980s to fast-food and full-service restaurants to offer a healthy alternative to fatty, high-calorie foods and to give the customers a wider choice of menu. In a study at the University of California at Davis, researchers watched 379 customers at salad bars in forty restaurants. They found that more than half of them—60 percent—touched or spilled food or behaved in other unsanitary ways.[18] Some people stuck a finger in the salad dressing, licked it off, and put the same finger back in another bowl of dressing. Others dropped bread on the floor, picked it up, and put it back in the container. Or they put their heads under the safety shields. People were even seen pushing uneaten lettuce from their plates back into the bowl of greens.

There are no statistics on illness from salad bars. One notable example, however, was the night before the 1984 Rose Bowl game, when nine UCLA players got sick, apparently from eating at a salad bar. Two were too sick to play, but the others recovered in time, and UCLA won.

Germs that cause food poisoning thrive in warm, moist protein foods, like chicken salad and cottage cheese.

I asked food inspectors what they would not order when they went into an unfamiliar restaurant. Most agreed that they would not order raw shellfish unless they knew that the product came from uncontaminated water. They would not order egg salad anywhere and would be hesitant about ordering any cooked salad such as potato or chicken salad. Many were even cautious about ordering ham sandwiches because, they said, cooked ham is a frequent source of foodborne infection.

A prominent cookbook author told me that she would never order chicken salad or lobster thermidor unless she knew the chef and he liked her. She said leftover chicken may be used for the salad, and the shells of lobsters may be taken from the plates of patrons who had whole lobsters, and kept around the kitchen for several days before being filled.

INSPECT THE RESTAURANT YOURSELF

Based on the opinions of the experts, here are the things you should look for when patronizing a restaurant:

- Is the outside clean? Are the bathrooms clean? Although other personnel may handle food, these factors are a good indication of whether the management insists on good sanitation.
- Are the dishes chipped? All equipment—including utensils and dishes—that touches food or drink should have a hard, smooth finish.
- Is garbage exposed? Are the counters and tables dirty?
- Are there flies or evidence of insect and rodent contamination?
- Are the food handlers smoking? Ashes from cigarettes or cigars and contamination from saliva are, of course, unsanitary.

• Is the restaurant in the basement? If it is, there is a greater possibility of contamination by flooding, sewage, and rats.

• Are the uniforms of the food handlers and servers clean? Do they wear caps to keep their hair from falling in the food?

• How do the waiters and waitresses set the silverware down? How do they serve the food? Are their fingers over and in everything?

• Are the glasses and silverware clean? Is there lipstick on the glasses or are there coffee grounds in the cup? (Water spots are not an indication of contamination.)

• Does the cream for the coffee feel warm? If it does, it is a good indication that it has been kept at room temperature and that temperature and time control are not observed by the management.

• Is the help coughing, spitting, or sneezing near the food?

• Are custards and cream-filled foods refrigerated?

• Are foods kept covered until they are served?

• Are the floors clean?

• In a restaurant other than a very small one, does a busboy rather than the server remove your dirty dishes? The server handling dirty plates may spread contamination to your food if busboys or proper sanitation are absent.

• If someone serves your food, does the server use a utensil instead of his hands?

• Are the menus dirty?

• Do the waiters or waitresses have sores on their skins or do they have improperly bandaged fingers if they have been injured?

• Are the salads served warm or wilted?

• If there is a salad bar, there should be a glass or plastic shield at face height (a sneeze guard) and a spoon, fork, or tongs for each container of food. See if the greens and vegetables appear to be fresh or wilted or discolored. Items like macaroni salad should also look fresh and not dried out. All food should be kept properly chilled or iced, and the salad bar should be kept clean. When a container of food is almost empty, it should be replaced.

THE CATERED AFFAIR

The catering business, health officials admit, is one of the weakest links in food-protection efforts in the United States. The majority of local and interstate caterers are not inspected and can operate without supervision.

Quoted in the first edition of this book, Vernon E. Cordell, then director of public health and safety for the National Restaurant Association, said that the proliferation of multiple-unit operations, franchised operations, and food services performed by management contractors had brought the food industry up against the problem of lack of uniform sanitation regulations.

The situation remains the same today. Instances of poisonings from all sorts of catered affairs are still numerous and involve large numbers of people.

In June 1989, eighty-six people were reported ill after a dinner held at the St. Demetrius Center in Carteret, New Jersey. The center is affiliated with the St. Demetrius Ukrainian Orthodox Church.[19] The dinner was organized by the church's men's club and attended by about three hundred. The food was purchased from commercial distributors and prepared by club members in the center's kitchen.

Eleven of the eighty-six had to be hospitalized. Six cases of *Salmonella* were positively diagnosed among them. Those who were sickened ranged in age from three to sixty. The complaints of illness included vomiting, stomach cramps, fever, and diarrhea. The *Salmonella* infection usually causes symptoms six to forty-eight hours after exposure.

The food served at the dinner included shrimp, roast beef, spare ribs, chicken, and manicotti. Most of the food was purchased from a wholesale food distributor. There were about fifteen people who prepared and served the dinner.

A spokesperson for the corporation where some of the food was purchased said that many of the same items had been sold to other groups and there were no complaints of illness.

The New Jersey Department of Health reported that *Salmonella enteritis* was found later in the chicken dish and kielbasa served at the dinner. That strain of *Salmonella* bacteria usually is associated with infections of eggs, chicken, and meat.

This case is typical of the type of catered affair that is involved in an outbreak of foodborne illness.

Current practices relating to this category of food service vary throughout the country. Some health agencies include such organizations in their inspections. Others exempt private clubs and church-affiliated and certain educational organizations from permit or license requirements and regular sanitary inspections. "When this is the case," the Public Health Service says, "a rather substantial segment of the population receives no official health protection in this area of food control."[20]

Some food inspectors suggest that a person who wants to give a private party or who is in charge of arrangements for an organization first get in touch with the local board of health to determine if the caterer has a license. Big caterers usually have good equipment, including temperature-control trucks, experienced help, and good sanitation know-how. But it pays to ask questions. In the meantime, after checking with the local health department, readers should see that potentially hazardous food is not exposed to improper temperatures during the party and that food is not contaminated by improper handling, either by the food handlers or by the guests.

VENDING MACHINES

Though sales of products from vending machines are now in the billions, vending machines, like catering establishments, are a weak link in the food-inspection protection program. However, today there are practically no reports of outbreaks due to food purchased in vending machines.

Walter Reed, director of public relations for the National Automatic Merchandising Association, the trade group of the vending and food-service management industry, said that when the first perishable beverages were dispensed in vending machines, the U.S. Public Health Service was asked to draw up a model code. "From that time on, our organization has taken upon itself to carry on extensive standards and education programs." Of the five thousand companies in the vending business, fifteen hundred belong to the organization and account for 70 percent of the volume.

He said the sales of vending machines have been on a plateau for ten to fifteen years. The big growth was between 1955 and 1975. By 1975, all the possible locations were saturated. These machines are highly competitive with fast-food places.

Between 1957 and 1982, the vending of potentially hazardous sandwiches, casseroles, and entrées grew from under $100 million to $704 million annually (about one billion units). During this time, one documented case of food poisoning (two victims) involving machine malfunction and two cases caused by foods brought to the machine with preformed toxins were reported.[21]

That's a pretty good record. Of course, I personally know of two cases that occurred in 1968 and that I wrote about in the first edition of *Poisons in Your Food*. Sandwiches purchased from a vending machine at a suburban New Jersey mall caused a manicurist and her client to become ill, probably from foodborne *Staphylococci*, since the onset was so quick after eating the food. The cases—as most cases—were not reported to the authorities.

Reed said newer machines are now being developed that are "user friendly." They tell you how much money you deposited. He said it is less likely today that machines will go out of order.

Candy machines are another matter. They are not inspected, and it is up to the owner of the place in which they are placed and the route people who stock the machines to keep products fresh.

What Can You Do About Vending Machine Safety?

"Nothing," say food inspectors. "It is a closed mechanism. You simply have to rely on the operator."

But why not post a sign stating when the machine was last inspected, just as is done in elevators? Why not a list of standards posted for the product the machine sells, and a visible temperature gauge? If the machine is supposed to dispense hot food above a certain temperature, why not say so, and have a thermometer that can be read by the buyer?

ORDERING A HEALTHY MEAL

Since the first edition of this book, there has been a great deal of information made available on the most common "poisons in your food"—fat, calories, and salt. Once you are satisfied with the sanitary aspects of the restaurant, here are some hints about how you can enjoy eating out and reduce the intake of those ingredients that may be deleterious to your health.

I am on a very low salt diet because of a hereditary condition. When I have more than a very small amount of natural salt in food, I become nauseated and dizzy and my blood pressure rises a few hours after the meal; if the salt load is very high for my system, I will suffer for two days from nausea, vomiting, and inability to work.

Now, while most people are not as sensitive to salt as I am, my experiences in trying to protect myself from a salted meal while eating out at restaurants, banquets, and business lunches have taught me a lot about the truthfulness and knowledge among restaurant personnel.

First of all, many of those involved in food service know that salt comes from a salt shaker or box, but they do not know that monosodium glutamate, soy sauce, teriyaki sauce, and most marinating sauces are high in salt. They do not consider the fact that fish can pick up salt from the salted ice on which it is kept or that salted butter is high in sodium.

While most restaurant personnel will do their best to help those of us on a special diet, some will lie and say the food has been prepared as we requested. They figure that we will never know the difference, and if we do, they will have been paid for the meal and we just won't come back to the restaurant.

You can increase your chances of getting food prepared a special way if you choose a restaurant that prepares fresh food after you order it, not before. There is no problem asking that your food be cooked without salt or saturated fat if the restaurant chef does the cooking. However, in a large percentage of eating places today, the restaurant buys frozen portions and defrosts each one when ordered.

If your restaurant menu is long, with a great list of choices, chances are your meal will have been pre-frozen and heated up for you.

The Center for Science in the Public Interest, a consumer group based in Washington, D.C., and several other consumer groups petitioned the FDA and the USDA for labeling of fast foods in 1986. Congress also considered legislation that would order the agencies to require fast-food ingredient labeling. If passed, such legislation would strengthen the already negotiated agreements between state attorneys general and major fast-food chains in seventeen states. These agreements call for the chains to provide consumers with brochures listing ingredients of foods upon request.

Most of the burger and chicken chains serve foods that are high in fat, calories, and salt.

Michael Jacobson, executive director of the Center for Science in the Public Interest, points out: "Without ingredient listings, how can consumers 'vote' at the cash register against Chicken McNuggets (which contain ground-up chicken fried in beef fat)? How can consumers avoid yellow No. 5, the allergy-triggering dye—found in some milk shakes and other fast foods—that the F.D.A. requires to be listed by name when used in packaged grocery products?"

Jacobson adds: "In truth, consumers would be upset if labels on restaurant foods revealed the presence of 'ground up chicken skin,' 'sulfur dioxide' or 'yellow dye No. 5.' And that's precisely the benefit of ingredient information. Its mere presence would drive some of the most nutritionally worthless products right off the market."[22]

If You Stop for Fast Foods

- If you must stop at a fast-food place while driving, order that sandwich or burger without the high-fat sauce.
- Instead of a milkshake, try a substitute orange juice or the low-fat milk most chains now sell.
- Try a salad from the salad bar, but not if you are allergic to sulfa or are worried about people touching your food before you do (see page 215).
- Skip the ice cream and opt for fruit.

Diet-friendly Restaurants

The American Heart Association (AHA) offers a large program to convenience restaurants to lower fat and salt in the foods they offer. The AHA is helping by urging restaurants and hotels to dish out reduced-calorie, low-fat, low-cholesterol, moderate-sodium meals. Local chapters of the AHA have embraced the program and carried it to community restaurateurs. (Check with your local AHA chapter.) Denise Rector, staff nutritionist for the Los Angeles "Dine to Your Heart's Content" program, claims that 165 area eateries—from fast-food franchises to fine French restaurants—are participating.[23]

But even if your favorite eating place isn't dieter-friendly, it's still possible to navigate around calories. Use common sense as your guide and follow this breakdown of eating suggestions offered by Rector:

- *Chinese and Japanese food.* While typically low in calories and saturated fat, they can be high in salt. Beware of soy sauce and monosodium glutamate in large doses.
- *Mexican food.* Avoid the cheddar and jack cheeses and sour cream. They're high in fat content.
- *Italian food.* Favor leaner meats like chicken and veal. Stay away from breaded dishes or those sautéed in fat. Pasta isn't too bad if you eat only a small amount.
- *French food.* "Nouvelle cuisine," Rector says, "is good because it skips the heavy sauces (of traditional French cooking). And since French chefs are generally skillful with spices, ask them to eliminate the salt. You won't even miss it."
- *American food.* Hamburgers are high in fat—between 22 and 30 percent fat, in fact. The AHA recommends only 15 percent per meal, at most. Play it safe with tuna salad, chicken, baked whitefish, boneless chicken breast, and barbecued beef from a top-round cut.

Rector cautions against large portions. "A six-ounce steak is better than a nine-ounce steak," she says. "You don't really have to eat all the food on your plate. Another way to control portion size is to order an appetizer as your main course. And, if you order something with sauce, ask to have the sauce put on the side so you can control the amount in your food."

Instead of ordering prime ribs, it is wiser to opt for chicken, veal, fish, or top sirloin. Request that your meat or fish be broiled, baked, or barbecued—anything but fried.

Eating on the Road

As far as food safety goes, the cleanliness of American "road" restaurants leaves much to be desired. Not only may the food be tasteless and greasy, the floors and tables may be littered.

The litter is from the patrons, but it's remaining where it was placed is due to lack of help cleaning up. The restaurants—which do a tremendous volume because they have captive patrons who travel the highways—don't seem to have a high regard for quality and cleanliness. After all, you must stop there and you are an out-of-towner who will probably not return, at least not for a long time.

Several federal food inspectors and I were discussing the hazards of eating in some restaurants while traveling by car. They pointed out that the FDA actually has legal jurisdiction over places along the highway because they can inspect food that is used in interstate commerce. They wondered whether it would not be possible for federal inspectors to give a "seal of approval" to tourist places that qualified, saying they were sanitary.

The value of such a seal is obvious, and if you think so too, and have had some bad experiences while traveling, you could encourage such a step by writing to your congressman.

Eating in Foreign Places

About one-third of the sixteen million travelers from industrial nations—including eight million Americans—will develop diarrhea or "tourista" each year when traveling.[24] The diarrhea comes on suddenly, usually during the first week of travel, though it may occur at any time during the trip or even after you go home.

Attack rates for traveler's diarrhea in high-risk areas such as Mexico vary between 20 and 50 percent. All of Africa; large stretches of the Far East, excluding Japan, Hong Kong, and Singapore; much of developing Latin America; and most of the Middle Eastern countries are in the high-risk group. Most of southern Europe and a few of the Caribbean islands, specifically Haiti and the Dominican Republic, are in the middle-risk group. Some other Caribbean islands, Canada, the United States, Australia, New Zealand, and northern Europe are considered low-risk areas, according to the National Institutes of Health–sponsored Consensus Development Conference focusing on traveler's diarrhea.

Since the illness is acquired through ingestion of feces-contaminated food or water, what can you do to cut down your chances of getting sick while traveling?

- Raw vegetables, meats, and seafood are high-risk foods.
- Tap water, ice, unpasteurized milk and other dairy products, and unpeeled fruit may increase the risk.
- Safe beverages include bottled carbonated beverages, beer, wine, hot coffee or tea, and water that's been boiled or appropriately treated with iodine or chlorine.
- In order of increasing risk are private homes, restaurants, and street vendors.

9 ⌐ Those Convenient New Foods

What is a *convenient food*?

If you take a potato, wash it off, stick it in the oven, and an hour later take it out and eat it—is that convenient?

If you take a box of instant mashed potatoes; measure a cup of water, salt, butter; boil the water; measure the amount of flakes in a cup and pour it in the water; stir in the milk; then scoop it out and eat it—is that convenient?

In the first instance, you get just the potato and whatever you wish to put on it—butter, sour cream, chives, yogurt, or cheese. In the second, you get mono- and diglycerides from hydrogenated soybean oil, sodium acid pyrophosphate, sodium bisulfite, citric acid, and BHA.

Since most women are working outside the home, and everyone leads a busy life, no one—except gourmet cooks and professional chefs—wants to spend much time preparing food.

Two-income households with microwave ovens and videocassette recorders are at an all-time high. Family members often eat meals while watching a movie or a previously recorded TV program. Because time is critical, convenience is an important factor in selecting foods. Food-service establishments and supermarkets are prepared to provide that convenience.[1]

Some food-service outlets have added automatic teller machines to make paying for a meal more convenient. In some outlets, a consumer may now patronize a food-service drive-through, punch in a bank account number and food item selections, verify choices on a computer screen, be presented with a bill on the screen, and press "O.K." to bill his or her account for the amount of the purchase. According to government seers, this trend will continue at least throughout the decade.[2]

But in addition to our *instant food,* we want *instant health.* And yet we pay higher prices for food that others have processed for us and we increase the risk of contamination. We also swallow a lot of additives that wouldn't be necessary if the food weren't processed. The potato example at the beginning of this chapter illustrates this.

In the 1940s, the average housewife spent about five hours each day preparing three meals for her family of four. In a *Parade* magazine survey in 1987, women said the ideal cooking time is thirty minutes or less and the men said fifteen minutes or less.[3]

We are in such a rush all the time that we act as if we wish oranges came with zippers. *The Wall Street Journal's* Sue Shellenbarger says that they will, figuratively speaking.[4] A government scientist has discovered that if a certain enzyme is injected under the skin of citrus fruit, the peel just falls away, leaving the fruit clean and undamaged.

Food processors presented us with seventy-nine hundred new food products in 1987, the year for which the most recent information is available, up from fifty-six hundred in 1985.[5] Because a product is labeled "new" does not necessarily mean it is better or in fact that it is really new. The word "new," vendors have learned, lures us into buying.

Our penchant for buying "new products" costs us money because it costs the processors money.

In the first edition of *Poisons in Your Food,* I quoted Dr. Abel Wolman, who wrote in an article, "Man and His Changing Environment," in the *Journal of Public Health:*

> The increase in the number and variety of processed foods is considered by some to be synonymous with a better and easier life. It seems to be assumed that most individuals for one reason or another are unwilling to accept foods in their natural

state. Hence, every conceivable effort has been made to modify color, taste, structural appearance, texture, stability, nutritive value and substitute commodities. Such successful efforts to supplement, modify and conceal nature introduces innumerable problems of identification, of evaluation, of control, and of assessment of long-term biological effects.

To the orthodox problems of biological hazards in food, industry has added the major issues of chemical, biochemical, physical, and other adjustments. The natural and artificially induced shifts in food habits, new methods of food technology, and the intentional and inadvertent use of additives find the health officer confronted with a baffling set of conditions unheard of even a decade ago. . . .[6]

No one in America wants to go backward. We want both convenience and an abundant choice of food. Yet we want it, and should have it, free of hazard, and it should be of good quality. Too often, we are not getting what we expect and pay for.

The purpose of this book is to help you make informed choices at the store and at the dinner table. Below are some of the ways in which convenience foods are prepared and the benefits and potential hazards.

SLOTTING

There are 30,400 supermarkets in the United States. Most of us now shop in them, and in recent years they have become like giant old-fashioned general stores. Some even include banks and post offices as well as drugstores.

Stores charge manufacturers for putting their products in the store—some would call it a "kickback" but supermarkets call it a "slotting fee." Some supermarkets institute "failure fees" as well.[7]

Many of us no longer make grocery lists at home, as we used to do. We now make about 66 percent of our shopping decisions in the store, up from 46.8 percent in 1977.[8] We buy "on sight." Therefore, sellers are emphasizing point-of-purchase advertising. But since there is limited space in the supermarkets for displays, we are going to be lured by "talking" carts that trigger a recorded sales pitch just as we pass a certain display. There are already videos, special-for-the-store broadcast programs with music *and* commercials, and food-sampling salespeople—all pushing a product.

Because of our harried life-style, we are letting supermarkets do more and more of the preparation of our meals, from salad bars to take-out dinners.

Since 1965, food spending in America has climbed 46 percent, according to the Agriculture Department. But during that period, spending on food to be consumed at home—purchased mainly from supermarkets—grew only by 20 percent. Spending on foods eaten away from home—at fast-food restaurants, delis, and other places that prepare food—shot up by 89 percent according to the USDA.[9] In order to be competitive, supermarkets are stocking twice as many products as they did in 1984 and are doing a lot of preparing for us.

Carry-out food is reported to be a $15 billion business. Supermarkets attract about $3.5 billion of this market, while small grocers, convenience stores, and delicatessens attract almost $2 billion.

The delicatessens within supermarkets are the fastest-growing sections, with gross margins averaging about 48 percent, while dry grocery foods are about 22 percent. Customers react differently in the deli than they do in other areas of the store. Perhaps it is a throwback to the days of Mom and Pop grocery stores, where human beings waited on you.[10]

We may not have choices about our parents or our taxes, but we do have choices about the food we select. And, as we said before, the object of this book is to provide information so that you will make better-informed choices.

Let's start with where and how we shop.

THE SUPER-SUPERMARKET

When you go into a supermarket, what do you look for? The items on your grocery list? The special bargains of the day? Few of us look for signs of good sanitation in any of the nation's more than 30,400 modern food stores.

The average supermarket invests thousands of dollars in temperature and humidity control to keep food in top condition. Yet physical damage to food products from breakage, bruising, and other mishaps that occur in warehousing, in delivery to retail stores, and in the stores themselves costs millions annually. About three-fourths of this damage occurs in the store, with employees causing about 60 percent of it and customers about 40 percent. Some of the damage is not recognized until after the customer gets the product home.

The Kings supermarket chain in New Jersey, an upscale operation, has its own corporate sanitarian, Gary Moore. He checks sanitation at the suppliers, the shelves in the store, the hot water, the cooking in stores, the displays, and even the trucks that deliver the food.

Most of us do not select our supermarket; the market selects us by establishing a store in our neighborhood. Fortunately, the majority of stores do a good job of food protection; but all have a problem in maintaining quality, and a few harbor sickness on their shelves.

Inspection of supermarkets, like inspection of restaurants, food-processing plants, caterers, and farms, is spotty and sometimes nonexistent.

I went into a brand-new, luxurious super-supermarket with Dr. Paul LaChance, associate professor of nutritional physiology at Rutgers University, New Brunswick, New Jersey.[11] There were wide aisles with thousands of products invitingly displayed. It looked like a housewives' shopping heaven to me. Yet Dr. LaChance showed me fish in broken plastic bags inadequately protected and refrigerated; chicken in packages that were perforated, with legs sticking out and juice dripping into the cabinet. (Shoppers were handling the chicken with their bare hands, pushing aside the packages.) Sliced bologna, inspected by a local health department, was two months old; honey jars were leaking; hams were unrefrigerated; potatoes had heart rot; meat was packaged so that the underside and sides were hidden from the shopper; processed foods were piled high, and some, such as dough and cheese pirogies, were soft instead of frozen.

In the years since, I have seen similar violations in supermarkets, particularly in the salad bars and the selection of rolls and other bin-type foods.

Dr. LaChance could read some of the mysterious codes on packages to determine their age.

"See this?" he said. "People believe the stores put the older products in front and the new products in back. They usually reach toward the back to select a package."

The product that Dr. LaChance had selected from the back was much older, according to the code, than the product in the front.

The following are the risks and benefits of having others process your food for your *convenience*.

SNACK FOODS

Supermarkets are filled with packages of potato chips, cookies, cheese bits, crackers, and all sorts of snacks that are usually salty, sugary, fatty, or dry.

The difference between a snack and a meal has blurred. Because parents are working and everyone in the family has his or her own agenda, the family meal where everyone sits down together is becoming extinct.

Robert Hilleque, publishing director of Harcourt Brace Jovanovich's snack group publications, including *Snack Food Magazine,* says, "About 60 percent of the population is 40 years old or younger, and they are snack food eaters who don't have the time or interest to sit down and eat three squares a day."

As Hilleque suggests, people are eating portable foods while on the run and then rewarding themselves for all their hard work by indulging in an expensive or high-caloric taste treat.[12]

Call it luncheon meat, deli meat, or cold cuts, those little see-through packages of sliced bologna, ham, turkey, and salami that you find on pegboards above supermarket meat counters are a boon to sandwich preparers who have little time to fuss over brown-bag lunches. Just slap a few of the round- or square-shaped slices between two pieces of bread (you don't even have to cut the meat), add a lettuce leaf and a tomato slice along with a hit of mustard or mayonnaise, and presto—a midday meal for under a dollar. Unfortunately, as with many quick fixes, there's a nutritional price to be paid. Many varieties of packaged cold cuts are high in fat. A full 84 percent of the ninety calories in a single slice of beef bologna, for instance (one slice in this case equals one ounce), comes from fat. And fat contributes 77 percent of the seventy calories in a one-ounce slice of salami. Of course, not everyone puts just one or even two slices into a sandwich, so those fat calories keep adding up. The American Heart Association says that we should limit the amount of fat to no more than 30 percent of our daily calories.

Those convenient deli meats are also high in sodium. Most of the cold cuts contain between two hundred and three hundred milligrams of sodium. Multiply that by three or four slices and you have one-third to one-half of all the sodium that should be consumed in an entire day, according to the National Academy of Sciences.

Even low-fat, low-salt versions of cold cuts may be higher in fat and sodium than is recommended for a healthy diet. For that reason, you should think about choosing cold cuts as an occasional change of taste rather than as standard fare (providing your physician does not rule against delicatessen items for you).

FRESH REFRIGERATED PRODUCTS

These processed foods are designed to offer the convenience of frozen and canned foods while providing homemade taste and appearance and, typically, are cooked just enough to ward off spoilage for a short period of time. As a further aid to freshness, they are often sealed in packaging that contains little or no oxygen, which can extend shelf life for several weeks.

As easy to prepare as frozen or canned products but boasting the freshness and eye appeal of home cooking, these products are known in the food business as "fresh refrigerated." They are the biggest thing to hit the industry since the microwave. Within the food industry as well as the FDA, however, there are growing concerns about these foods that include everything from pizza to filet mignon. According to many experts the new packaging and processing techniques potentially offer a breeding ground for an array of dangerous bacteria, most notably those causing botulism.

As Alix M. Freedman, a staff reporter, said in the *Wall Street Journal,* "Ironically, consumers may be courting food poisoning in their haste to get the looks and tastes of mother's kitchen without any of the bother."[13]

"This is the unexplored side of the fresh, refrigerated foods business that could have very adverse consequences for consumers," says Joseph Hotchkiss, associate professor of food science at Cornell University. "The science and technology are going into developing the new products, but virtually no one is doing research to find out what the risks are and how to control them."[14]

Consumers are beginning to clamor for the new products. A Michigan State University study estimates that fresh prepared foods now account for about $500 million of the $450 billion U.S. food market. Industry analysts estimate that sales will grow a rapid 14 percent a year.

What accounts for the success? People are sick of canned and frozen goods that are processed to a pulp, food experts say, and they are less concerned about the dangers of fresh refrigerated foods than they are about the dangers associated with food additives.

"They perceive the risk from fresh refrigerated foods only as a bellyache," says Mona Doyle, president of Consumer Network, a research company in Philadelphia. "And to them, a bellyache is better than the possibility of cancer from a lifetime of preservatives and additives."[15]

But scientists are concerned that some dangerous bacteria may not be killed during the initial precooking characteristic of fresh refrigerated foods. And the microorganisms that cause botulism can flourish in an oxygen-free environment—precisely the kind of packaging used for many of the new products.

Moreover, the most dangerous bacteria—*Listeria, Yersinia,* and botulism—don't always make food smell or taste spoiled (see chapter 6).

"What is really alarming about fresh refrigerated foods is that consumers could do everything right and there could still be a problem, particularly if the product wasn't heated again," says Lloyd Moberg, head of the microbiology department at General Mills, Inc.[16]

Sous-vide, a technology imported from France, has sparked the most controversy because of the fear of botulism. The technique, which reached the United States in the early 1980s, calls for sealing fresh raw ingredients in an oxygen-free pouch, which is cooked under precisely controlled heat and moisture conditions. The pouch is then chilled and ultimately given a quick cooking before landing on a diner's plate. The appeal is the enhanced flavor, the preservation of freshness for three weeks or more, and, as a growing number of U.S. restaurateurs report, decreased labor and food costs. The technology also holds out the promise of virtually kitchenless restaurants, which can just reheat pouches produced off site.

Big food processors are getting into it. Almost every major food processor, as of this writing, either has products in development or being test-marketed. They are trying to work out the logistics for delivering a wide range of refrigerated fare to sprawling American markets. They also must convince consumers that although fresh refrigerated food costs more than cooked meals from the delicatessen section of the supermarket, it is worth it. They must also convince us that they have erected sufficient barriers to prevent potential hazards.[17]

FROZEN FOODS

What's the situation with frozen foods today?

Because of their high water content, most foods freeze easily at temperatures between 25°F and 32°F. Although each food has a specific freezing point, quick freezing takes place in thirty minutes or less. If freezing is rapid, damage to the food is reversible. Slow freezing permits large, uneven crystals to build up; these puncture the food cells and make the food mushy when it is defrosted.

Though 50 percent of the live organisms are killed in frozen food in six months and 75 percent in one year, this does not mean that the food is safe. It may have been handled in an unsanitary manner and may have food toxins and other contamination.[18]

At the Frozen Food Packers National Association meeting in Chicago, former FDA commissioner George P. Larrick said:

Routine bacteriological controls are not sufficient to detect potentially pathogenic microorganisms which may be present in raw ingredients.

Pesticide residues in frozen foods are a problem requiring unique controls where raw agricultural commodities of a perishable nature are purchased.

An ever-present problem, both for the frozen-food packer and the FDA, is the care employed in adding just the right amount of direct food additives for which there are tolerance limitations. There is a basic assumption in the use of these that the food manufacturer will take the necessary precautions to avoid misuse.

The really dangerous frozen food is that prepared by the independent small-time merchant who wants to freeze something he makes himself. Delicatessens and specialty stores do it, most of the time without proper equipment and without any inspection at all. In such cases, one man's frozen dish may truly be another man's poison.[19]

CANNED FOODS

When Napoleon had his hand in his shirt, he may have been hiding the first can of food.

All eighteenth-century soldiers traveled in peril from their diets of putrid meat and other inferior food. In order to improve the condition of his fighting men, Napoleon offered a prize of twelve thousand francs for the invention of a method of food preservation for his army. A confectioner, Nicolas Appert, observed that food cooked in sealed bottles remained unspoiled as long as the container remained unbroken. Appert won the prize in 1809. By 1820, the first commercial canning plants were operating in the United States, and by 1840 canning was common throughout the country.[20]

Considering the number of cans produced annually, the record of the American canning industry has been remarkably good. Commercially canned food may be stored almost indefinitely under proper conditions. Sealed cans are heated during the canning process to destroy undesirable organisms. Although acid foods may react eventually with the tin and iron in the can to cause off-flavors, such a taste is not an indication of spoilage. Canned foods should be stored in cool places to retard such reactions. There is a considerable loss of vitamins when canned vegetables and fruits are stored in a warm place.

One of the biggest problems with canned foods is not bacteriological contamination but the addition of high levels of salt. In recent years, a number of "low-salt" products have come on the market, but they are more expensive.

Drying

Drying food to preserve it is as old as man's discovery that the sun can stop decay.

In the 1700s, people put their food near the fire, or else spread it in thin layers in direct sunlight, to hasten drying it. In 1795, two Frenchmen named Masson and Challet made an important improvement in the process of drying when they built a dehydrator in which air heated to about 105°F was blown over thinly sliced vegetables.

The first dehydrated instant foods, however, are credited to the United States Army Quartermaster Corps. In World War II, the corps came up with instant mashed potatoes that tasted very much like wallpaper paste. During the war the Quartermaster Corps issued a contract to industry to improve dried potatoes. The improvement was made, and a host of other dehydrated products was developed, including eggs, milk, and some vegetables. The processing reduced shipping weight, eased storage problems, simplified distribution, and enabled soldiers to carry their rations with less effort in the field. Though these World War II products still lacked quality and were difficult to rehydrate, they were the forerunners of today's many dried convenience products.

Before 1950, most dehydration was done in cabinets or tunnels with forced blasts of air at high temperatures to remove water. Such methods caused damage to the product. Today, vacuum-drying in cabinets is used for prune cakes, apple powder, and potato granules.

Spray-drying and drum-drying are also used for dehydration. Improvements in heating methods, water removal, and temperature control make spray-drying and drum-drying techniques applicable to more foods in greater volume. Coffee, tea, soup mixes, fruit solids, and vegetable purees may be spray-dried.

A newer method is puff-drying. The product is partially dehydrated by circulated hot air; then it is exploded (puffed) by a gun. The food is finish-dried in heated bins to withdraw the last traces of moisture. By using this method, the United States Department of Agriculture has puff-dried carrots, beets, blueberries, and apple pieces.

Studies on a significant number of samples of various dehydrated fruits and vegetables have shown that very few, if any, of them are sterile. Little information is available concerning the significance of microbial populations found in these products.[21]

A combination of both freezing and dehydrating techniques is "freeze-drying." This is a process in which moisture is removed from the food while it is in a frozen state. The advantage of freeze-drying is that the water is removed in a manner that does the least physical damage to the food itself. Freeze-dried foods now include soups, casserole dishes, fruits for cereals, and coffee. They retain their flavor, aroma, and stability much better than air-dried foods.[22] One critical problem with freeze-dried foods is that they absorb water more rapidly than do other dried foods. Therefore, they require special packaging and handling. These facts, plus the higher cost for water removal, mean that the cost of freeze-dried products is usually high.

MICROWAVE

More than 80 percent of households in the United States will have microwaves by 2000, up from 66 percent in 1987, according to a National Family Opinion study. A standard oven was used to prepare only 15 percent of meals in 1987; 47 percent of them required the use of a stove's burners. In 1989, microwaveable products generated $750 million in sales.[23]

Microwaves have also become a fixture in the work place, where penetration has been estimated at 70 percent and there has been a big push for zappable lunch products. Microwavable foods are also convenient to distribute and store, a plus when freezer space is at a premium.

Microwaving may also have a nutritional advantage. Bacon from the microwave may be better for you than bacon fried in a pan. Chemists from the National Center for Toxicological Research (NCTR) in Jefferson, Arkansas, say microwaved bacon retains all of its pleasurable features but probably lacks most of the potentially cancer-causing nitrosamines formed during frying.

"The method of cooking nitrite-cured meats such as bacon affects the level of nitrosamines in the cooked product," Barbara Miller reported at the 194th national meeting of the American Chemical Society in 1989.

Nitrosamines are a class of chemicals that are known to cause cancer in some laboratory animals. Researchers have known for years that nitrosamines can form when nitrites are exposed to direct high heat, such as in frying. Meat packers use nitrites in bacon, lunch meats, and other products for curing, improving color, and preserving.

Barbara and Dwight Miller and Stanley Billedeau of NCTR cooked bacon in a skillet and in a microwave oven and measured resultant levels of two nitrosamines—n-nitrosodimethylamine and n-nitrosopyrrolidine—both listed as carcinogens by the Environmental Protection Agency. The Millers found higher levels of both in the skillet-cooked bacon. They also found that levels of these carcinogens were higher in residual fat on the cooked bacon than on the cooked meat itself.

"At forty-five seconds in the microwave on its highest setting, we found no nitrosamines at all," Barbara Miller said. But when cooked for 75 seconds, n-nitrosopyrrolidine showed up at levels of 5 ppb (parts per billion). It is unknown if this level is dangerous to humans, but similar levels administered to rats have resulted in tumors, she said. In the skillet-cooked bacon, both types of nitrosamines were detected, sometimes at levels of over 20 ppb.[24]

Scientists theorize that the lower levels of nitrosamines in microwave-cooked bacon meat are due to the form of cooking energy.

Microwave energy probably is not as likely to convert nitrites to nitrosamines as is direct thermal energy, they say.

The Millers, who use a microwave oven to cook bacon at home, said that microwaved bacon tastes every bit as good as skillet-cooked bacon. "Given the choice, I would cook bacon in the microwave," Mrs. Miller said.

Retailers and producers are, of course, still concerned about safety issues. One case of botulism could destroy the business.

IRRADIATION

When food is irradiated, it is loaded onto a conveyor belt and passed through a radiation cell where it is showered with beams of ionizing radiation produced by high radioactive isotopes. The radiation can inhibit ripening and kill certain bacteria and molds that induce spoilage, so that food looks and tastes fresh for up to several weeks.

Irradiation of food would seem to be the answer to all problems of foodborne disease and quality loss. When the government proposed radiating food, a brochure was published by the Atomic Energy Commission, Division of Technical Information, describing the process. It promised:

Oranges as sweet and juicy as if just picked . . . strawberries firm and free of mold—yet all many miles and weeks away from harvest. How is it possible? They've been *radiation-pasteurized* . . . exposed to low levels of nuclear radiation.

Bacon, ham and chicken that haven't been near a refrigerator in months are fed to hundreds of soldiers who find them the equal of normal fresh meat. How? They've been *radiation-sterilized* . . . exposed to levels of radiation high enough to kill bacteria . . .[25]

The process does not make food radioactive, nor does it change the food's color or texture, in most cases. Does it destroy nutrients? After food has been exposed, does it create radiolytic products that may cause genetic damage? Is irradiation less dangerous than some of the other chemicals added to foods as preservatives? These questions are being hotly debated.

The FDA requires foods that have been irradiated to say so on the label and to display an international logo, a flower in a circle.

Other than canning, radiation processing is the only original—that is, nonnatural—method of preserving food. The amount of radiation to be delivered depends upon the food itself and the result desired. If the goal is prolongation of shelf life, or storage time, a pasteurization dose, generally 200,000 to 500,000 rads, is sufficient. If the food is to be sterilized for long-term storage without refrigeration, the required dose is between 2 million and 4.5 million rads.

Even lower doses of radiation—4,000 to 10,000 rads—stop potatoes or onions from sprouting. Twenty thousand to 50,000 rads kill insects infesting food. Doses of 200,000 to 400,000 are highly effective in extending the refrigerated storage of fresh fish up to thirty days. Bacon and other pork products, chicken, and beef can be packaged and then irradiated at 4.5 million rads, resulting in sufficient preservation to permit a year's storage at room temperature.

Irradiation could save us money by stopping food spoilage; it could also help underdeveloped countries without adequate refrigeration and food distribution.

The FDA gave a green light to food irradiation on April 15, 1986, for treatment of fruits and vegetables, herbs and spices, white potatoes, and wheat and wheat flour. (Irradiation was already allowed for the treatment of pork.) Under the 1986 regulations, radiation doses of up to 100,000 rads—a dose of radiation equivalent to more than thirty million chest X rays—can be used to treat fruits and vegetables, and up to 3,000,000 rads can be used to disinfect spices and herbs.

The FDA's approval of food irradiation has prompted outcries from legislators and other concerned citizens who consider the FDA's action to be overly hasty and scientifically unfounded.[26]

Under the FDA regulations, the product has to be labeled "treated with radiation" or "treated by irradiation." Originally, the FDA proposed that irradiated foods be labeled "picowaved." Foods that contain irradiated ingredients but have not themselves been irradiated do not have to be labeled. For example, cakes containing spices that have been irradiated do not have to be labeled nor does frozen pizza or foods served in restaurants, dormitories, hospitals, prisons, and the military.

The safety of food irradiation has not been proven. Studies have found kidney and testicular damage, as well as chromosomal damage in animals fed irradiated food. Also, the possibility of risk of cancer from consuming irradiated food cannot be ruled out since studies have shown an increase in tumors in mice and rats fed irradiated food.

A study in the 1960s at Cornell University showed that eating irradiated sugar can produce the same results as irradiation directly applied to the cell. Scientists experimented with carrot tissue and coconut milk . . . both high in natural sugars. They bombarded them with cobalt 60, causing radiation-induced cell mutations in both foods. Moreover, the chemicals produced by sugar breakdown in the foods were seen in transfer radiation effects into the cells of fruit flies, resulting in stunted growth and chromosome damage. All living cells contain sugar, the report emphasized, and human beings may suffer similar consequences from long-term consumption of irradiated food.[27]

There are also many studies maintaining that irradiated food is wholesome.

Perhaps radiation will prove to be the answer; perhaps we shall go back to older methods. In fact, United States Department of Agriculture researchers reported at the 1968 meeting of the American Institutes of Biological Sciences in Urbana, Illinois, that ultraviolet light (the same as that of the sun) can kill 99 percent of the harmful bacteria in maple syrup. They said control of bacterial growth by ultraviolet light irradiation is "simple, inexpensive, leaves no harmful additives, yet is 100 percent effective."

NATURAL OR ORGANIC FOODS

When Eve handed Adam the apple, it may have had a worm in it, but it didn't have any pesticides, wax coloring, or chemical fertilizer. We all know the consequences of taking a bite of the first apple, but what about the aftereffects of today's fruit?

The proof that people are worried about this problem is the phenomenal growth within the past year of health-food stores across the country; in these stores, people are paying from two to three times as much for an "unadulterated" apple as they would for one from the corner supermarket.

Perhaps you can reduce the amount of poisons in your food by buying products from a "natural" food store. The problem is that you are really fighting a losing battle. As the chapter on pesticides in this book relates, bug killers, sprayed from planes and even by hand, get into the streams and into the air. If you drink water and breathe air, you are absorbing pesticides. The same is true about other chemicals in the air and water.

So-called food faddists, however, who have been promoting the use of natural food, additional vitamins, and restrictions on the use of additives, have lived to see the day when many of their contentions have been proved in scientific laboratories.

At the National Conference on Cancer of the Colon and Rectum in San Diego, California, in January 1971, a British cancer specialist, in a speech to nearly a thousand delegates, said that colorectal cancer could be a product "of the modern Western diet of over-refined foods and confections."[28]

Many natural-food enthusiasts had been blaming cancer and other ills on the American diet. At the conference on cancer, Dr. Wendell Scott, clinical professor of radiology at Washington University, St. Louis, Missouri, stated:

> If the addition itself be without intrinsic nutritional value, but somehow necessary to assure that the full nutritional properties of the foodstuff reach the consumer, and there is no substitute, rigorous standards are required to establish what level of risk is acceptable. Lethality is quite out of the question, but an incidence of one reversible untoward incident per 500,000 consumers, for example, may be an acceptable risk.

> If, however, the additive offers no form of nutritional value but is present to enhance flavor or texture, the public is entitled to assurance that such addition is quite without hazard, viz., failure to detect metabolic or physiological alterations, abnormalities of development, mutations, or neoplasia. By

failure is meant that the odds against such unwanted effects be at least greater than a million to one at ordinary levels of intake, with no detectable chance of lethality whatsoever. We sadly lack a data base for making such statements concerning most additives or many drugs. . . .

This is not to urge that food additives be removed immediately from all food preparations but, rather, that we embark upon the extremely large effort required to obtain such data. . . .

Fresh, organically grown, or "additive-free" foods at health-food stores, to this consumer, do taste better. Nevertheless, we should not have to pay three times as much to obtain food without unwanted chemicals. Most chemicals added to our food are added for the benefit of the seller, not the buyer.

You do have a choice in where you shop and what you buy. You also have a responsibility to be alert and informed; when you see something wrong, you have a responsibility to report it. Most store managers want to please their customers and will go to great lengths to do so.

WHAT YOU CAN DO
Check Sanitation

- Is the store clean? Are the floors dirty?
- Are the shelves messy?
- Are the people who work in the store untidy-looking?
- Are there bathrooms available for customers? For the help?
- Are the bathrooms clean and properly equipped with soap and paper towels?

Check Refrigeration

- Meat is supposed to be refrigerated at 28°F to 38°F; produce and nonfrozen dairy products at 35°F to 45°F; ice cream at −12°F.
- Are hams and other processed foods that require refrigeration under refrigeration? How about eggs? They should be refrigerated too.

- Check the condition and temperature of packages. Are the contents in cardboard cartons that block cold air?
- Are the products overloaded in the cases? Does the thermometer in the case register 0°F or below? (Remember, the thermometer is usually in the coldest spot in the case, so there ought to be a good margin of safety.)
- Is there evidence of leakage about a package of frozen food? Your purchase should be frozen solid, with none of the contents adhering to the outside of the package.
- If large quantities of ice crystals are present on the inside walls of a package of frozen fruit or if the fruit is somewhat shriveled, it is suggestive of thawing and subsequent refreezing or long-time storage. If there is considerable ice formation on the bottom of the package of dry packed fruit, the item may have been thawed and refrozen.

Check Precooked Frozen Foods

Appearance and odor may help to tell you, once the food is defrosted, that it is not of good quality. They may indicate that the product has fermented during processing by reason of a slow freeze or that it has been allowed to thaw. A dry, bleached surface is indicative of improper packaging, excessive storage periods, or widely varying temperatures in frozen storage.

Check Canned Foods

Don't look for bargains. Never buy an unlabeled or a dented can. Acid foods may react eventually with tin and iron in the can to cause an off-flavor. This undesirable flavor is not an indication of spoilage. However, it is better to be safe than sorry. The deadly botulinus sometimes causes off-odors and off-tastes. Canned food should be stored in a cool place to retard off-flavors. There is also a considerable loss of vitamins when canned vegetables and fruits are stored in a warm place.

Check Jars

Never buy a jar that is sticky or leaking.

Check Produce

Look at the bottom of the lettuce. If it has a brown instead of a white ring, it is old; this may be an indication of the practices of the management.

Think Twice About Buying Something New

According to Jean Judge, food-marketing specialist at Rutgers College of Agriculture and Environmental Science, "The customers who typically buy new products are usually those who most frequently reject the traditional housewife's role in food purchasing and preparation and thereby set the buying patterns for new products.

"They are most likely to be those who live in the urban areas of the Far West or Northeast, are well educated, represent families wherein the housewife is employed outside the home, have medium high incomes. Typically, families with young or school-age children are more likely to use new products, especially convenience items, than families without children."

Manufacturers of products know that an item is not profitable for more than two to five years; some items are profitable for a shorter period of time. Yet, the word "new" does not necessarily mean better. For example, Consumers Union found that a new food package that allowed the consumer to put a package of bacon into a toaster for instant cooking could cause a severe shock.[29] New vacuum-sealed envelopes in which smoked fish was packaged allowed botulinus spores to multiply, and a score of persons who bought the packages died of botulism.

This does not mean that food processors and vendors should stop trying to make improvements and developing conveniences for Americans. It does mean that each "new" product should be thoroughly tested for safety first. It's best not to rush out to buy something new; rather, hesitate long enough to see if it is really of good quality, and safe.

Once you get home with your packages, if you find something wrong with a purchase, report it to the store manager. If the situation is not rectified, alert your local board of health. You owe this to yourself, your family, and your fellow shoppers.

Demand adequate inspection of food processors, supermarkets, and other vendors of food.

Remember, your best protection remains your own skill and education as a buyer.

10 ~ Some Questions and Recommendations

In the first edition of *Poisons in Your Food,* I wrote:
It is not the purpose of this book to be sensational, nor is it to attack farmers, food processors, restaurants, government agencies, or any specific group. Its aim is not to point out that illness and death have resulted from what we eat, although this is certainly true. The author has no desire to hinder technology in its development of new and better means of preparing, packaging, and serving food.

The goal of this book is to raise questions. Have we, like unsupervised children with beginners' chemistry sets, unrestrainedly poisoned ourselves and perhaps our descendants?

In a report to the secretary of health, education, and welfare by the Task Force on Environmental Health and Related Problems, dated June 1967, it was pointed out that "We know something of air pollution, but we know little about the potential hazard of 500,000 to 600,000 synthetic chemicals and other compounds on the market today. We know something of water quality but little of the effects of trace metals. . . .

"An individually acceptable amount of water pollution added to a tolerable amount of air pollution, added to a bearable amount of noise and congestion can produce a totally unacceptable health environment. . . .

"It is entirely possible that the biological effects of these environmental hazards, some of which reach man slowly and silently over decades or generations, will first begin to reveal themselves only after their impact has become irreversible.

"Not only have we overwhelmed many of nature's processes for environmental stability; we have misused, without knowing it, biological processes upon which the preservation of life depends. By allowing tiny amounts of pesticides to enter our waters, we have set in motion processes that can lead to the destruction of birds that feed on fish that feed on plants that draw the pesticides from the water. Our ignorance of the consequences of our deeds may be innocent, but it is ignorance we can no longer tolerate."

But today, we are still tolerating it.

The same weakness we had in protection then, we have today. In fact, there are even greater gaps. There are fewer personnel and less money and more to be done by the agencies that protect our food supply. We have, furthermore, millions of newly vulnerable AIDS victims and the aged, all with compromised immune systems.

The Delaney Amendment, which once stood as a bulwark against the addition of known cancer-causing agents to our food, has quietly crumbled.

The Delaney Food Additives Amendment, Public Law 85-929, was passed on December 6, 1958. The law specifically states that *no additive may be permitted in any amount if the tests show that it produces cancer when fed to man or animals or by other appropriate tests.*

Food and chemical manufacturers and even the Nutrition Council of the American Medical Association attacked the Delaney Amendment at the time of its passage. The AMA Council on Nutrition urged either repeal or revision of two clauses in the Food Additives Amendment and the 1960 Color Additives Amendment. Both clauses prohibit the setting of tolerances for the use of cancer-causing agents in food.

"These clauses could prohibit the addition of certain essential nutrients to foods in any amount if the substance was shown to cause cancer. Technically, these clauses contribute nothing to the safe use of food additives since any hazardous use of an additive is already prohibited in the general provision of the food additives amendment."[1]

The secretary of health, defending the clauses, said: "No one really knows how to set a safe tolerance for substances in given foods when those substances are known to cause cancer when added to the diet of animals.

"Eminent scientists, including those on the National Academy of Sciences Food Protection Committee, state that no one, at this time, can tell how much or how little of a carcinogen would be required to produce cancer in a human being or how long it would take the cancer to develop."[2]

The National Academy of Sciences Food Protection Committee, while agreeing that low doses of a known carcinogen have been applied in small amounts to mouse skins without cancer developing, stated:

"The possibility exists that doses at 'no effect' levels do in fact exert carcinogenic effects but that the effects are too weak to detect with the numbers of animals feasible for routine testing. Such a possible effect, though extremely weak, might become evident in a large population such as, for example, the population potentially exposed to food additives in our culture. There is also the possibility of synergistic effects among substances present in the diet and of an individual susceptibility to carcinogens, although little is known about these factors."[3]

Despite the fact that no one can determine what amount of a cancer-causing agent causes cancer, the FDA has decided to literally break the Delaney law.

In a speech on the subject of safety assessment, given in 1984 before the International Life Sciences Institute in Japan, Sandford A. Miller, director, Center for Food Safety and Applied Nutrition, Food and Drug Administration, said:

In 1982, the FDA published an Advance Notice of Proposed Rulemaking announcing its intention to apply a new policy for assuring the safe use of food additives and color additives that contain minor amounts of carcinogenic chemicals.

Prior to this notice, the Agency, with few exceptions interpreted the FD&C Act to ban the use of any additive found to contain even minor amounts of carcinogenic chemicals.

Since the publication of the notice, the FDA has applied the principles of this risk assessment policy to a number of food additive and color additive issues on a case-by-case basis. Three of these have involved noncarcinogenic color additives for drug or cosmetic use *in which there are identifiable levels of the cancer-causing agent p-toluidine (made from coal tar). Another represents an application of this policy to an (indirect) food additive used in food-packaging materials.* (Emphasis added.)

A second broad policy involving risk assessment has concerned the use of animal drugs in food-producing animals. According to Miller, the FD&C Act contains a Delaney clause prohibiting the approval of animal drugs that induce cancer when ingested by a man or animal. However, in contrast to the food additive or color additive anti-cancer provisions, this one includes the so-called DES proviso (named after diethylstilbestrol, an animal growth hormone), excepting those carcinogenic drugs that leave "no residue . . . in any edible portion of such animals . . ." This exception prompted the FDA to propose to define the "no residue" standard by means of the sensitivity of the analytical method used to determine the presence of the substance. The sensitivity of the detection method is tied directly to the quantitative risk assessment for the substance in question (i.e., the level presumed "nondetectable" is defined by the estimated level of risk it presents). Thus, risk assessment has been used as a means by which assays for carcinogenic residues (both drugs themselves and their metabolic products in the food-producing animals) may be evaluated for safety under the animal drug anticancer provisions of section 512.[4]

Did you understand that last paragraph? In other words, now that the FDA has instruments sensitive enough to detect minute amounts of cancer-causing agents in foods, it will decide how much of a cancer-causing agent will be permitted in food, including the meat we eat.

Among the cancer-causing agents the FDA has set tolerances for, despite the Delaney Amendment, are aflatoxin (a mold), dioxins (highly toxic synthetic chemicals), and PCBs (a class of very toxic chemical substances used in a wide variety of industrial processes) in foods and lead acetate used in hair coloring.

Miller went on to say that the new "risk assessment" for decision making has been successful: "Ranging from the essentially no-risk philosophy embodied in the Delaney clause of the Food Additive Amendments to the more flexible risk-benefit component of the Toxic Substances Act, U.S. law has attempted to encompass a wide variety of philosophies in the use of risk assessment."

Today, the fact remains, however, that neither Miller, the FDA, nor the National Academy of Sciences—no one, as yet—knows how much of a cancer-causing agent causes cancer, so how can they set a "tolerance"?

HOW MUCH DOES THE FDA KNOW?

Does the FDA know all the food additives—intentional and unintentional—added to our food?

Although officially the FDA claims to know the additives used throughout the food industry, FDA researchers report that it is impossible to check all the small manufacturers. Efforts have been made through the years to have food manufacturers register and provide the information, but as yet there is no law requiring them to do so. In fact, food manufacturers—with the exception of those who make baby foods and low-acid canned goods—do not have to register with the FDA. How can the FDA really know what is put into food if it doesn't know that a manufacturer even exists?

Does the FDA know the true manifestation and number of adverse effects of food additives?

Since the first edition of this book appeared, the FDA established the Adverse Reaction Monitoring System (ARMS) in 1987.

Linda Tollefson, D.V.M., M.P.H., chief, Clinical Nutrition Assessment Section, Center for Food Safety and Applied Nutrition, in a letter to the author, explained:

The Adverse Reaction Monitoring System (ARMS) was developed in an attempt to identify adverse reactions to food products and additives regulated by the FDA. Although food and color additives undergo extensive safety testing before approval for marketing, it is not feasible that preapproval testing will uncover all potential adverse effects. Acute/subacute injury surveillance activities are needed to continually assess hazards associated with consumer exposures to foods and food and color additives. The ARMS was designed to retrieve and process data related to adverse health effects associated with specific foods or food additives and to help ensure the continued safety of newly approved food products and additives.

The ARMS is concerned with spontaneous reports of adverse reactions from consumers, and as such, is a form of *passive* surveillance.[5]

This means that the FDA does not go out and find adverse reactions but waits for you or anyone else who has an adverse reaction to report it. Then, if it is severe enough or common enough, the FDA will investigate.

Tollefson went on to say: "Reports describing severe reactions and specific case-defined groups are investigated by FDA field personnel. This involves interviewing the complainant or a close family member; interviewing the attending physician, if possible, and obtaining medical records; and if applicable, analyzing samples of the food suspected to have caused the reaction."

Tollefson noted: "Because of limitations of a passive surveillance system, the data generated from the ARMS are only used to assess the *likelihood* that a problem exists with a particular food product or additive." Definitive statements as to the probability of cause and effect between the reported symptoms and the implicated food additives are not made because of the inherent limitations of information gained from spontaneous reports from consumers.

She said among other problems in identifying a troublesome additive even when the food and the adverse reactions are both common is that there is no information about the prevalence of the adverse effects because no one has informtion about the exact number of people who consume the product in question or how many of them suffer ill effects after eating it.

Tollefson said the only way to find out this information would be to have a controlled study, such as a food allergy survey of a representative sample of the population.

"Reporting of adverse reactions will always be incomplete, due either to underascertainment or underreporting, and the degree of incompleteness will be unknown and variable. Underascertainment refers to the fact that most consumers and many physicians fail to recognize an adverse event as being related to a food additive or food product. In particular, serious reactions are more likely to be reported even if they occur less often than mild ones, and reactions which occur shortly after using a product are more likely to be associated with the product. Therefore, the serious and often rare symptoms which occur shortly after using a product are more likely to be detected by a spontaneous reporting system than the more common or delayed symptoms.

"Underreporting," she said, "refers to the failure by the consumer or physician to report an adverse event to a regulatory agency for a variety of reasons, even if they associate the reaction with a particular food product or additive. On the other hand, mass media attention can artificially inflate reporting rates. In addition, a critical population mass may be necessary and use of the product widespread in order to generate sufficient data to indicate if a problem indeed exists."[6]

ARMS is a good start in the attempt to find the true incidence of adverse reactions to food additives. It needs to be funded and it needs our cooperation. If you have an adverse reaction, you or your physician should report it to the FDA.

Milton Z. Nichaman, M.D., D.S., and R. Sue McPherson, M.S., at the University of Texas Health Science Center in Houston, believe that *active* epidemiological studies can also provide more information about food additives. They point out: "Adverse reactions to foods are a public health problem. However, the extent of this problem remains unknown because of a lack of information regarding the prevalence or incidence of these reactions in the general population.

"Clinical medicine focuses primarily on diseases in individuals whereas epidemiology replaces the individual focus with a population focus."[7]

Epidemiology seeks to describe the distribution of disease in a population to: person, place, time.

As a result, epidemiologists can then hope to predict the number of disease occurrences, affect the distribution of disease through prevention, and explain the cause of the disease.

The Texas researchers said, "The current body of literature concerning adverse reactions to foods contains only a small number of studies designed to address the issue of prevalence of these reactions. Because of numerous methodologic constraints in the study designs, very few studies actually present data that can be extrapolated to the general public."

In another attempt to gather information on food additives and their safety, the FDA's Bureau of Foods has set up a computerized data bank. Priority Based Assessment of Food Additives (PAFA) attempts to keep track of changes in dietary patterns of society as well as the development of new and important knowledge of potential toxic effects that can be associated with any additive or group of additives.

PAFA has in its data base 1,586 substances out of the 3,000 known to be added to our food supply. Alan Rulis, Ph.D., heads the program.

This, too, is a good start, but it leaves 1,414 food additives about which little or nothing is known. Furthermore, the data base has only the information published in the literature. No one is actually testing additives specifically for the data base.

Of course, ARMS and PAFA would not be very effective in citing cancer-causing agents since cancer may take from two to forty years to develop. Thus, epidemiological studies are badly needed, such as the ones cited on farmers and pesticides in chapter 2.

Why is the cancer rate different among populations?

There is now scientific consensus that about 80 percent of cancer cases appear to be linked to the way people live their lives. For example, whether we smoke, the foods we eat, and certain industrial pollutants all affect the likelihood of our getting cancer.[8]

The role of diet in the cause and prevention of cancer is particularly important. In fact, the most comprehensive review to date estimates that 35 percent of cancer deaths may be associated with dietary influences.

Colon cancer is one type of cancer that is linked to diet. Few people realize that colon cancer is over three times more common in the United States than it is in Finland; that colon-cancer deaths in Connecticut are more than 70 percent higher than in Utah; that the colon-cancer death rate in the American black population has almost doubled in the last thirty years and now equals that of the white population; that the frequency rate for colon cancer among Hispanics in Los Angeles is only two-thirds that of other whites in Los Angeles; or that people living in Florida—even in areas of the state where 40 percent of the population was born in the northeastern United States—have substantially less colon and rectal cancers than do their northeastern countrymen. These are just a few examples of cancer differences that may be linked to diet.

The possibility of preventing colon and rectal cancers is suggested not only because of the high prevalence in the United States compared with other countries with different eating habits, but because of evidence that risk may be lowered substantially within an individual's lifetime by changes in diet. The National Cancer Institute believes the main factors increasing colon-cancer risk are too much dietary fat and too little dietary fiber.

We must ask ourselves why the United States has a cancer death rate of 216.6 per 100,000 population for males, why Japan has a rate of 194.3, and Israel a rate of 157.

Is it heredity or diet? It has been shown that when Japanese women have moved to the United States, their rate of breast cancer is low among the first generation, who follow the Japanese diet, and gradually increases in mothers and granddaughters as the American diet is adopted.

Do certain food ingredients—synthetic or natural—promote cancer?

Vincent DeVita, Jr., M.D., director of the National Cancer Institute, made a statement during U.S. Senate Appropriation Hearings on March 5, 1986, and U.S. House of Representatives Appropriation Hearings on March 11, 1986:

> Cancer cells are renegades. They exert lethal effects by growing out of control, but they appear to be immature, somewhat confused cells, aberrantly using the same genetic mechanisms established for normal growth and development. The new biology allowed researchers to tap into this genetic machinery at the heart of the cell and find minute, but critical, differences in genes of normal and cancer cells. They discovered oncogenes involved in transforming healthy cells into cancer. The counterparts of these genes, proto-oncogenes, are involved in normal growth and development. It has long been thought that cancer is a multistage process with intricate circuits and switches, working at different points of disease progression and at different times. Some substances serve as initiators that start but cannot finish the cancer-causing process without the help of promoters. Most promoters cannot work in cells that have not been initiated. With new technology, we can study the genetic switches which trip the cascade of events that control growth and development or lead to cancer. Although cancer is over 100 different diseases [sic], we now feel certain they share some basic mechanisms that set off the disease and have already exploited some of these data at the clinical level.

Recent research in cancer etiology has focused on how promoters work, because interfering with promotion may yield results by preventing cancer in persons exposed to initiators and offers the best hope in our lifetime of reducing cancer incidence. Powerful evidence already exists that this approach works—for example, curtailing wide use in the 1970s of the "promoter" estrogen, which caused uterine cancer in postmenopausal women.

Saccharin is a tumor promoter. We need research to determine tumor promoters in our diet and stronger laws to remove them once they are identified.

Are there neurotoxins in our food?

The Chemical Industry Institute of Toxicology (CIIT), Research Triangle Park, in Triangle Park, North Carolina, founded in 1974 by the chemical industry, is working to develop new neurotoxicology tests. Dr. M. E. Pruitt, now a retired vice-president of the Dow Chemical Company and CIIT's first chairman, said: "By 1974, it became clear to many of us that much more toxicological data was needed on most chemicals."[9]

A CIIT position paper, released in April 1987, said that many of the questions asked in 1974 were still unanswered.[10] Among them:

- Which chemicals are dangerous, especially over long periods of time?
- How much exposure is too much?
- Are certain combinations of chemicals (or combinations of chemical exposure and certain elements of a life-style, such as smoking or drinking) more dangerous than others?
- How can we identify in advance, rapidly and economically, chemicals that may cause problems?
- And, most important, how can the sum total of our observations of chemical toxicity be rationally compiled and analyzed so that we can make informed decisions about the benefits of a compound versus its risk?

The CIIT paper noted that among the "priority public issues" on which the current research program is focusing are:

- Concern about reproductive and developmental or other adverse health effects from exposure to chemicals present in air, water, or food.
- The "emerging issue" of neurotoxicity.

Hugh A. Tilson, Ph.D., head of the neurobehavioral section of the National Institute of Environmental Health Sciences, Laboratory of Behavioral and Neurological Toxicology, in North Carolina, maintains that routine tests for neurotoxins should be included when screening food additives.[11]

"We are not involved in the setting of regulations but provide data that might be used by an agency to determine whether there is toxicity present or not," he explains. That data doesn't have to be used. The FDA currently has no guidelines for neurotoxicity tests, and they should have. Dr. Tilson says there are simple and inexpensive tests—for example, studying the grip strength of animals and motor activity—that could be done by technicians who now do other tests on animals.

Dr. Tilson points out that aspartame was extensively tested with routine toxicology tests and was shown to be a fairly innocuous substance. But researchers need to take an animal population that is predisposed toward seizures and see if the chemical exacerbates an already existing propensity. If the chemical does the same in the human population predisposed to seizures, then people should be warned about ingesting it.

Dr. Tilson says that red flags about aspartame do exist. These are anecdotal reports about some people who say they experienced discomfort and some who have reported actual seizures.

Is additive testing adequate?

The federal government asked the National Research Council of the National Academy of Sciences to evaluate the current tests and to determine further testing needed to evaluate the safety of food additives and other chemicals. The NRC drew the following conclusions:

- When judged against current standards for toxicity testing, 92 percent of the tests being used were inadequate.
- Of eighteen standard tests used, only one—the oral administration in rodents test—was judged to be adequate. The other seventeen standard tests that were used either were not done adequately or were not done at all for 67 to 100 percent of the food additives.
- As far as food additives were concerned, a large variety of other tests were found to be needed such as chronic studies, inhalation studies, and more complex studies such as neurotoxicity, genetic toxicity, and effects on the fetus.
- There is no toxicity information available at all for 46 percent of the additives and only 5 percent of the food additives had enough test information to make a complete health hazard assessment possible.

The fact is that a large percentage of the food additives have not undergone long-term testing, which is one of the great problems in determining chemical safety. Cancer, for instance, may take twenty years to develop in humans and often more than two years to develop in animals. Right now, the FDA determines long-term safety of a food additive from studies in rats that live from eighteen to twenty-four months. However, researchers point out that laboratory animals are in a nonnatural, sterile environment and that in two years, 70 to 90 percent of them would be dead anyway and only two or three would be left for evaluation. Therefore, these long-term tests may have invalid assurances of safety.

There have been thirty-five and a half widely used food additives removed since 1972 because of an association with cancer or toxicity. (FD&C Red no. 3 was partially removed from use in 1990 because it causes thyroid tumors in rats.[12])

What happens when additives combine?

Another great problem with testing additives is how they interact with each other and with the sixty-three thousand other chemicals in common use today.[13] In 1976, the *Journal of Food Science* carried a report on a small-scale attempt to determine the extent of the problem. When three additives were tested one at a time on rats, the animals stayed well. Two at a time, the rats became ill, and with a three-additive combination, all the animals died within fourteen days.

How well are our government agencies protecting us from harmful food or food of poor quality?

Because of lack of personnel and money, the agencies, no matter how well intentioned, cannot adequately do their job today.

Even if the FDA did have the personnel available to adequately monitor all that needs to be monitored, and they found serious lapses, what could they do?

Unlike most govenment regulatory agencies, the FDA does not have subpoena authority either to summon witnesses or to require firms to divulge pertinent records. It has requested this investigative authority to allow it to do a better job of protecting the American public. To date, the request has been denied by Congress.

A ray of sunshine has broken through since the first edition of this book was published. The FDA is now allowed to fine offenders up to $500,000 instead of the previous $1,000 per count. The increase was the result of the Criminal Fine Enforcement Act of 1984, which provided new fines for federal law violations perpetrated after January 1, 1985. The following fines are applicable for each offense:

- Up to $100,000 for a misdemeanor by a corporation or individual not resulting in a death.
- Up to $250,000 for a misdemeanor by an individual that results in death, or for a felony.
- Up to $500,000 for a misdemeanor by a corporation that results in death, or for a felony.

The maximum imprisonment for a misdemeanor under the FD&C Act remains a year for each offense.

With respect to foods, the administration must have considerably more authority to assure adequate protection of the public health. The department must be able to evaluate the synergistic effects of food additives so that the consumer is protected from threats that cannot be detected by the separate analysis of the individual food additives. This means evaluating the total of the toxicological effects of a mixture.

Furthermore, the administration must have, as it does not now, adequate authority to inspect and evaluate the processing of foods to make certain that their safety is not impaired through the effects of a process that may or may not involve the use of additives.[14]

In my tours of food-processing, -handling, and -retailing establishments, I learned that federal and local inspectors first sign in with the management. A health officer explained to me: "We do it out of courtesy. Most people have nothing to hide and if they do, they can do it so well, the notification of our presence wouldn't make one bit of difference. . . ."

The shortage of qualified personnel for the purpose of food protection, ranging from physicians to local inspectors, is acute. For instance, the FDA is desperately in need of "qualified specialists to review and evaluate scientific and clinical data." Unfortunately, our government is offering $15,000 to $20,000 less in salaries than these scientists can earn in private industry.

When you offer low pay for a difficult job, chances are you are setting the stage for corruption. This was shown dramatically when half the New York City health inspectors were indicted for corruption in 1988 (see page 214).

Government agencies have also been hard-pressed to keep abreast of new developments because the resources for food protection programs have not kept pace with the rates of technological change or population growth. The government's programs are largely based on visual inspection for gross defects in products, facilities, and procedures where food is processed, stored, or prepared for serving. These techniques are not adequate to cope with centralized manufacturing, mass distribution, mechanical dispensing, and commercial catering of prepared products.

The job of the FDA is complicated by a crucial overlapping of functions with the Department of Agriculture. Thus, the FDA does not deal with pesticides and herbicides and other toxic materials that contaminate food because the Department of Agriculture does.

The FDA lacks prestige and has such a modest salary ladder that it has great difficulty attracting promising, well-trained employees, especially physicians.

The FDA has approved chemical agents despite inadequate testing, only to withdraw them later on the basis of new studies. Some of the pressure has come from other countries. Oil of calamus, for example, was used for years in fruit, chocolate, root beer, vanilla, and so on. It was withdrawn in 1968 because it was found to cause malignant tumors in animals. NGDA, used in shortening and other such products, was removed from the "generally safe" list after Canada banned its use there and created pressure for its ban in the United States.

In 1992, when the United States of Europe become a reality, will some of our foods be banned from sale because they do not meet European standards? As we have seen, our meat has already been refused because of our use of hormones in beef.

And there are no ways for the consumer to know what has been added. The law requires only that labels say an artificial coloring, flavoring, or preservative has been added. The label does not have to list them. If a person is sensitive to those things, there is no way for him to know what not to eat.

The FDA has been and still is understaffed, underfinanced, and demoralized. The situation there has not improved. It may be that the agency is ungovernable.

Although they are rare, there are criminals in the food business, from the shady buyers of contaminated foodstuff to truck hijackers to shellfish bootleggers, and we are not being adequately protected from them.

The subject of chemical additives in our food has perhaps received more attention than many other aspects of food safety. Yet relatively little has been done about it.

Since certain food additives, just as certain pesticides and other chemicals, have residual properties, the imposition of setting tolerances for these substances will not eliminate their threat to health.

Are imported foods safe?

The FDA has a handful of inspectors on import duty.

The rapid increase in containerization—the practice of shipping huge packages with many different items in each—is another new headache for food inspectors. For instance, when such containers arrive in the United States, should they be opened at the port of first arrival or be shipped to the inland point near the ultimate destination?

The FDA and the USDA are not permitted to open private mail, and yet investigators have told me that this is the way some contaminated foodstuffs get into the United States.

What happens to vitamins in processed foods?

As unbelievable as it may seem, we do not have accurate methods for determining what happens to the vitamins in our foods from the time they are harvested or processed until the time we eat them.

We cannot answer the question of whether severe heat and dehydration processes in the preparation of precooked and easy-to-prepare "convenience" foods affect the nutritional quality of our food.

In 1970, the Department of Agriculture announced that researchers had found that milling and bleaching wheat for bread and cakes destroys 90 percent of vitamin E and 85 percent of vitamin B.

Vitamin E is the body's natural protector against peroxidized or rancid fat. It is necessary to keep blood, arteries, and the heart in good working order. It is also destroyed in freezing, so that those who eat all their meals as TV dinners or who take all their vegetables from the freezer may be lacking vitamin E.

This is just one of many uncertain areas in nutrition research. We do not know the effect of a pregnant woman's diet on the fetus. Scientists previously believed that the placenta, which provides nutrition for the growing embryo, protected it from harmful chemicals in the mother's system. Now it has been discovered that not only does the placenta not protect the child, it may even concentrate and increase the harmful substances delivered to the fetus.

Do pesticides cause cancer?

The studies linking farmers suffering from cancer with their use of pesticides as well as the other cases of cancer linked with pesticide use mentioned earlier have answered that question—yes, they do. In what doses and over what period of time are still uncertain.

Are there significant amounts of pesticides still in our food when we eat it?

The answer is yes, as you can read in chapter 2. Again, how much is significant over what period of time is still not known.

A reevaluation of the entire use of pesticides should be undertaken.

Nonchemical methods of pest control should be encouraged by means of greater financial support.

Can natural foods contain toxins?

Again, the answer now seems to be yes. Increasing evidence that the cycad plant causes malignancy is being gathered. Some common foods contain hazardous levels of toxins in special situations. For example, green potatoes have high levels of glycoalkaloids, including solanine. Common foods can become toxic if prepared in nontraditional ways; one example is the consumption of raw red beans, which can cause intestinal upsets. Some foods eaten in excessive quantities can cause upsets—for example, lima beans, cassava roots, millet sprouts, and chick peas. Knowledge and moderation are the best protection against such toxins.[15]

Has tracking of foodborne illness improved since the first edition of Poisons in Your Food *was published?*
No, it has deteriorated. Questions about the effects on our health of what we eat and drink are almost endless. No one knows—and there are no figures available on—the true incidence of food poisoning in the United States because so many incidents go unreported or because deaths from food poisoning have been wrongfully attributed to other causes. Furthermore, the money for personnel and computer support has faded and thus statistics are gathered every five years instead of every year. That's a disgrace and a danger to public health!

What are some of the answers to problems in food safety?
If this book raises many questions, it also presents some obvious answers. I asked an FDA official what he would do if he had unlimited power to improve the safety of our food supply:
"I would like to see more involvement of top management in industry," he said. "What happens in a food or drug plant is that an inspector goes in and gives the report to the plant manager. The plant manager doesn't want to be the bearer of bad tidings, especially when the boss holds him responsible. Many top executives do not know what is going on in their own plants."
From government experts, university scientists, physicians, and others concerned with what we eat, here are recommendations for steps that should and could be taken without delay:

INCREASED KNOWLEDGE ABOUT FOOD

We need research programs to produce new basic knowledge about both natural and processed foods in relation to health. These should include, but not be limited to, the study of new production, processing, and marketing methods as they may affect public health.

We need more food science departments in institutions of higher learning in the nation. There are at present thirty-nine, and many of them are acutely understaffed and underfinanced. One food science professor told me that his department was so short of funds, they could not even subscribe to technical journals. In relation to the size of the food-processing industry, as we have already indicated, the number of trained food scientists who are now graduating or whom one may expect to see graduating in the years ahead is woefully small, particularly when one considers that many graduates assume academic or governmental, rather than industrial, positions.

One of the most cheering events that happened since the first edition of *Poisons in Your Food* appeared is the establishment in the late 1980s of the National Center for Food Safety and Technology. Located at the Illinois Institute of Technology (IIT), it presents a new concept—a center where academia, industry, and government pool their resources and work together to achieve the ultimate goal: "ensuring the continued safety and quality of our food supply."

The sponsoring organizations include the Institute of Technology, IIT Research Institute, the University of Illinois at Urbana-Champaign, and the U.S. Food and Drug Administration. Attending the center are visiting scientists from industry and academia.

If it works out—and it is too soon to tell if it will—the center will represent a giant step taken not only toward preventing problems but toward training future personnel who will protect our food supply. Staff scientists include experts in biology, toxicology, food chemistry nutrition, polymer chemistry, and process engineering. They can work together on the safety and effectiveness in the production processing, packaging, storage, and distribution of foods.

Physicians Need to Study Nutrition

The Food and Nutrition Board of the National Academy of Sciences reported that 60 percent of medical schools offer less than twenty hours of instruction in nutrition,[16] and yet few today would deny that proper diet is one of the most important health-maintenance factors.

CHEMICALS

Nitrites, which are salts or esters of nitrous acid, should be banned from all products immediately.

Immediate efforts should be made to survey the true amount of nitrates, which are salts or esters of nitric acid, in our water and food, and immediate steps should be taken to further reduce and eventually eliminate such residues.

CHEMICALS AND ANIMALS

The use of antibiotics and hormones in feed should be reevaluated. They have proven to be a detriment to both animals and humans and eventually an economic liability, not an asset. Some control over the administration of medications to ill animals should be established. Since farmers are not trained in veterinary medicine, diagnosis and therapy should be left to veterinarians.

FROZEN FOODS

A complete survey of frozen foods should be made, from the time of slaughter or harvesting to their preparation, packaging, sale, cooking, and appearance on the dining room table.

No truck should be permitted to transport frozen food without adequate refrigeration and a graph to determine temperature control from the time of pickup to the time of delivery.

New safeguard devices, such as the strip of tape that shows whether a package has been defrosted, should be developed and used.

BETTER USE OF MANPOWER

There should be a coordinated inspection of food, from growth and harvesting to the manner in which it is recommended that it be cooked. Overlapping and gaps in the use of manpower should be abolished.

Pay scales should be raised, and an effective, concerted effort should be made to interest young people in food protection services.

FISH

Fish should be inspected under the law, and stricter standards should be made and enforced.

The American shipping industry should be revitalized by private and government subsidies for new equipment and by restrictions on imports.

SOME OBSERVATIONS

Our methods of growing food are not as efficient as those of the Japanese. If they were, California could feed the nation.

Our trucking is not as adequate as Britain's; there, temperature graphs are required by law.

Our regulations governing pesticides are not as strict as Germany's.

Our food doesn't taste as good as French food does.

The food we eat on earth is not as safe as the food we provide for our astronauts; in space, upsetting the delicate balance between man and microbes could cause disaster.

But our supply is wondrous in its abundance and variety. Our level of sanitation is above that of many countries, where diarrhea kills off a large percentage of the child population.

For all-around quality, the American food supply is the best in the world—but it could be much better—and safer!

11 Home Fires and Freezers

No matter how well our food is grown, manufactured, inspected, warehoused, and retailed, if we don't handle and prepare it properly ourselves in our homes, we and those we love will suffer from foodborne illnesses.

Based on the advice of experts in all fields, here are methods for protecting the food you buy:

- Do your grocery shopping last, and head immediately for home.
- If you cannot go home immediately, take a cooler in your car and place the perishables in it.
- Always wash your hands before preparing food and after touching meat, and before touching produce that will not be cooked.
- Don't allow anyone with an infection, including yourself, to prepare food.
- Purchase—and use—an accurate thermometer in your refrigerator.
- Keep the inside of the refrigerator clean. Wash it at frequent intervals.
- Keep the areas around the motor and refrigerating unit clean. Lint and dirt on these parts cut off the supply of air, causing the

motor and the refrigeration unit to overwork, thus reducing their efficiency.

- Check the gaskets around the doors. Be sure that they are flexible and prevent the cold air from escaping.
- If your refrigerator is not self-defrosting, check the cooling area frequently and defrost it. A buildup of ice on the cooling coils acts as an insulator, and the refrigerator will not work as well as it should. When the ice builds up to one-fourth of an inch, it is time to defrost.
- Store foods in small, shallow containers. The more surface that is exposed to the cold, the faster the food will cool. Keep foods covered, so that the food particles from the shelf above will not fall into the food stored below. Allow space between food containers and between all foods and the walls of the box.
- Never cover the wire shelves of the box with paper or foil, as this cuts down on the circulation of air within the refrigerator. Never stack foods on top of each other.
- Because bacteria grow between 45°F and 120°F, refrigerate food immediately after it is cooked. This means all foods, including roasts, stews, leftovers, broths, and puddings. Any delay will allow bacteria to grow more rapidly.
- If much hot food must be refrigerated, cool it first. Place the food in a shallow pan and set the pan in cold water. Be careful, of course, not to let the water mix with the food. Unless the cooling unit is overloaded, it is perfectly safe to put hot things in today's modern refrigerators.
- Keep hot things hot. Use a meat thermometer to check pork and other meats. In general, foods should be kept hot at a temperature above 140°F.
- If you have been in a traffic jam or some other incident that has delayed you in getting newly purchased food home to your refrigerator, be sure that temperatures reach 165°F to 170°F in the center of the food that is being cooked.
- Keep eggs in the refrigerator.
- Store bread, in its original wrapper, in a bread box or refrigera-

tor. Bread keeps its freshness longer at room temperature, but in hot, humid weather, it is better protected against mold in the refrigerator.

- Store flours, cereals, spices, and other grains at room temperature in tightly closed containers that keep out dust, moisture, and insects. During the summer, buy such foodstuffs in small quantities only.
- Store butter, fat drippings, and margarine in tightly wrapped or covered containers in the refrigerator. These products should be used within two weeks. Don't let them stand for long periods at room temperature.
- Keep all homemade salad dressing in the refrigerator. Purchased mayonnaise and other ready-made salad dressings should be refrigerated unless used within a few days.
- Cold cuts should be stored in the refrigerator and used within three to five days.
- Store ham, frankfurters, bacon, bologna, and smoked sausage in the refrigerator in their original packaging. Uncooked cured pork may be stored longer than fresh pork, but the fat will become rancid if it is kept too long. Bacon should be eaten within a week for best quality, a half a ham in three to five days, a whole ham within a week. Ham slices should be wrapped tightly and used in a few days.
- Ground meats, such as hamburger and fresh bulk sausage, are more likely to spoil than are roasts, chops, or steaks because they have been exposed to contamination from air, food handlers, and mechanical equipment. Store them loosely wrapped in the coldest part of the refrigerator and use them within one or two days.
- Although some food scientists say you can keep leftover stuffing from cooked fowl separate from the bird in the refrigerator for one or two days, it is best to throw it out.
- Fresh milk and cream should be stored in the refrigerator at about 40°F. Milk and cream are best stored only three to five days. Keep them covered so they won't absorb odors and flavors from other foods.

- Keep dry milk in a tightly closed container and reconstituted dry milk in the refrigerator.
- Keep hard cheese in the refrigerator. Wrap it tightly to keep out air, and trim away any mold that forms on the surface of the cheese before use.
- Store soft cheeses in tightly covered containers in the coldest part of the refrigerator. Use cottage cheese within three to five days, and others within two weeks.
- Keep synthetic mustards, milks, and puddings in the refrigerator.
- With few exceptions—such as potatoes, dry onions, hard-rind squashes, and eggplants—keep vegetables in the refrigerator. Discard any vegetables that are bruised or soft or that show evidence of decay or worm injury.
- Wash all fruits and vegetables before eating them.
- Store honey and syrups at room temperature until opened. After their containers have been opened, honey and syrups are better protected from mold in the refrigerator.
- Store nuts in airtight containers in the refrigerator. Because of their high fat content, nuts require refrigeration to delay rancidity.
- After a jar of peanut butter has been opened, it should be refrigerated.
- When freezing food, package it so no moisture can enter. Containers should be leakproof.
- Records should be kept so that you know what foods are on hand and what foods need replenishing in the freezer. This will keep you from storing food too long.
- If a power failure develops in your freezer, or if the source of power is temporarily shut down, keep your freezer closed to retain the low temperature. Frozen foods in a fully loaded freezer will often stay frozen for as long as two days; in a half-filled freezer for about a day.
- Thawed fruits can be safely refrozen if they taste and smell good.
- Other foods that have thawed spoil more quickly. Special care

is necessary in handling vegetables, shellfish, and cooked foods that have thawed or partially thawed.

- Freezer burn—white dried-out patches on the surface of meat—won't make you sick but will make meat tough and tasteless. To avoid it, wrap freezer items in heavy freezer paper, plastic wrap, or aluminum foil. Place new items to the rear of the freezer and old items to the front, so that they'll be used first. Dating freezer packages also tells you what to use first.
- Once a food has been thawed, it is wise to use it as soon as possible and not to refreeze it.
- Do keep frozen foods, especially poultry, in the refrigerator during thawing. If you have to speed up the defrosting of a turkey, place it under running *cold* water. Roasts, including turkeys, may go into the oven frozen; just increase the roasting time.
- Don't defrost meat and poultry on the kitchen counter. Bacteria can multiply rapidly at room temperature, and besides, chances of contaminating the counter and, subsequently, other food are increased.
- Do keep meringues, custard-filled éclairs, synthetic custards, doughnuts, and pastries in the refrigerator. Take them out just in time to serve.
- Do chill main-dish salads for large groups in shallow bowls or on trays in the refrigerator, and keep an eye on their temperature during the meal.
- Do keep sandwiches or sandwich fillings in the refrigerator until served. Covering sandwiches with a damp cloth is not recommended, since bacteria grow especially well under such circumstances. In fact, sandwiches should not be made the night before. Cooked meat next to damp bread makes an excellent breeding place for bacteria.
- Do keep a separate pan for washing dishes. Dishwater should be 130°F or above. Be sure that the rinse water is clean and hot and that the towels are clean.
- Don't empty your pet's dish in the same sink you use for washing dishes and preparing the family's food. Your pet's dish

may well be contaminated with harmful bacteria. In fact, avoid allowing pets in areas where food is being prepared.

- Don't use or buy canned foods if any of the following signs are present: bulging of the top or bottom of the can; dents along the side seams; any sign of seepage, off-odor, or foaming when the can is opened; any unusual milky quality of liquid.
- Don't buy or eat salads, especially mayonnaise-based salads, that have not been or are not refrigerated.
- Don't use leftover food if discoloration, off-odor, or mold is apparent. Any food that has not been refrigerated below 45°F may be considered to be slightly spoiled. Recook any leftover food that has been kept in the refrigerator thirty-six hours or longer. The cardinal rule of food safety at home is: *When in doubt, throw it out!*
- It is more important than ever before—as you have read throughout this book—that meat and poultry be thoroughly cooked. Use a thermometer inserted into the thickest part of the meat, avoiding fat and bone.
- Don't interrupt cooking, because partial cooking may encourage bacterial growth before cooking is completed.
- When cooking frozen food allow one and a half times the period required for nonfrozen food.
- Thoroughly reheat leftovers. Cover the dish to retain moisture and to be sure the food is heated all the way through. Bring gravies to a rolling boil before serving.
- Never leave food out for more than two hours.
- Make sure that sponges, cloths, and towels that are used to wash and dry dishes and utensils are kept clean. Bacteria can multiply in moist and dirty materials.

The last pages of this chapter tell you where to obtain more information and where to report problems.

Remember that we consumers have the weakest lobby in Washington. Our own education is our strongest safeguard against poisons in our food.

COLD STORAGE OF MEAT AND POULTRY*

Time limits? Because you can't tell exactly how long meat and poultry will last when you get them home, this chart gives short, conservative storage times. You may be used to keeping food longer, but following the chart will help protect you from food spoilage—what you risk with long refrigeration—and from taste loss—what happens when food is left too long in the freezer.

Product	Refrigerator (Days at 40°F)	Freezer (Months at 0°F)
FRESH MEATS		
Roasts (beef)	3 to 5	6 to 12
Roasts (lamb)	3 to 5	6 to 9
Roasts (pork, veal)	3 to 5	4 to 8
Steaks (beef)	3 to 5	6 to 12
Chops (lamb)	3 to 5	6 to 9
Chops (pork)	3 to 5	3 to 4
Hamburger, ground and stew meats	1 to 2	3 to 4
Variety meats (tongue, brain, kidneys, liver, and heart)	1 to 2	3 to 4
Sausage (pork)	1 to 2	1 to 2
COOKED MEATS		
Cooked meat and meat dishes	3 to 4	2 to 3
Gravy and meat broth	1 to 2	2 to 3
PROCESSED MEATS (Frozen, cured meat loses quality rapidly and should be used as soon as possible.)		
Bacon	7	1
Frankfurters	7†	1 to 2
Ham (whole)	7	1 to 2
Ham (half)	3 to 5	1 to 2
Ham (slices)	3 to 4	1 to 2
Luncheon meats	3 to 5†	1 to 2
Sausage (smoked)	7	1 to 2
Sausage (dry, semidry)	14 to 21	1 to 2
FRESH POULTRY		
Chicken and turkey (whole)	1 to 2	12
Chicken pieces	1 to 2	9
Turkey pieces	1 to 2	6
Duck and goose (whole)	1 to 2	6
Giblets	1 to 2	3 to 4
COOKED POULTRY		
Covered with broth, gravy	1 to 2	6
Pieces not in broth or gravy	3 to 4	1

Cooked poultry dishes	3 to 4	4 to 6
Fried chicken	3 to 4	4
GAME		
Deer	3 to 5	6 to 12
Rabbit	1 to 2	12
Duck and goose (whole, wild)	1 to 2	6

*From *The Safe Food Book,* USDA Food Safety Inspection Service
†Once a vacuum-sealed package is opened. Unopened vacuum-sealed packages can be stored in the refrigerator for two weeks.

FOR FURTHER INFORMATION AND WHERE TO REPORT A PROBLEM

The Meat and Poultry Hotline
USDA-FSIS, Rm. 1163-S
Washington, D.C. 20250
Telephone: (202) 472-4485
(Staffed 8 A.M. to 4:30 P.M.
EST)
TDD for hearing impaired:
(202) 447-3333

FDA Office of Consumer
Affairs
HFE-88, 5600 Fishers Lane
Rockville, MD 20857
Telephone: (301) 443-3170

U.S. Department of
Commerce—NOAA
National Marine Fisheries
Service
3300 Whitehaven Ave.
Washington, D.C. 20235
Telephone: (202) 634-7458

Cooperative Extension Service
For questions on food handling,
nutrition, and storage.
Listed in your local phone book
under county government
or state university.

Public Citizen Health Research
Group, 2000 P St., NW,
Suite 700
Washington, D.C. 20036

Public Voice for Food and
Health Policy
1001 Connecticut Ave., NW,
Suite 522
Washington, D.C. 20036

Center for Science in the Public
Interest
1501 16th St., NW
Washington, D.C. 20036

Clean Water Action Project
317 Pennsylvania Avenue, SE
Washington, D.C. 20003

12 ~ Understanding Labels and Food-Freshness Codes

You don't eat your own words—you "eat" the food processors' words—"lite," for example, or "natural" or "portion."

The labels on food products are supposed to tell us what is in the container and how much it will nourish us. About 55 percent of food includes some nutritional labeling.

Ingredients are listed in descending order according to weight. But you can't tell how much of a particular ingredient is used— although if you are buying beef and noodles, the package will say "beef and noodles" if there is more beef and "noodles and beef" if there are more noodles. Furthermore, there are many names for sugar and salt, so that if you add up all the sugars in a product, for example—sucrose, dextrose, corn syrup, and honey—sugar might be the main ingredient in the product, even though it is not listed first.

Nutrition information is required on a food label when a manufacturer adds a nutrient to it or when a claim is made for the product, such as "now contains fewer calories." Protein and certain vitamins and minerals may be added by manufacturers to make a food more nutritious (called *fortification*) or to restore nutrients lost in processing (called *enrichment*).

As you read in chapter 9, many ingredients—such as specific flavorings and food colors—do not have to be listed on the label.

276

Senator Howard Metzenbaum's recipe for better health has one major ingredient: a heaping measure of accurate nutritional information.

"For far too long, we Americans have been shopping in the dark," the Ohio Democrat said in 1989 as he and other lawmakers joined together to support the proposed Nutrition Labeling and Education Act.[1] Metzenbaum added that the mandatory uniform labels required by the bill would eliminate what "are at best confusing—at worst, downright deceptive" labels voluntarily provided by many food manufacturers and processors.

The legislation had the support of twenty-three nutrition and health organizations, including the American Heart Association, the Center for Science in the Public Interest, the American Cancer Society, the American Dietetic Association, the American College of Physicians, and Public Voice for Food and Health Policy.

Representatives from most of the groups praised the bill for recognizing long-standing scientific research and educational efforts linking nutrition with deadly illnesses such as heart disease and cancer.

The bill would:

- Make nutrition labeling mandatory on processed food sold in the United States.
- Require disclosure of certain essential pieces of information, including the amount of fiber, fat, and cholesterol, and the type of fat.
- Use recommendations from the National Academy of Sciences to improve the format of labels and provide comparative context for the information.
- Provide clear and definite standards governing claims and statements involving such terms as "lite" and "cholesterol-free."

Metzenbaum criticized the Food and Drug Administration for moving slowly on the issue.

Senator John Chafee (Republican, Rhode Island) echoed that concern, pointing out that it had been sixteen years since any fundamental change had been made in the way foods are labeled.

While processed food labels need improvement, nutrition labeling is not required on meat and poultry products.[2]

Products bearing special claims such as "low calorie" and "low sodium" are exceptions; processors must explain what these claims mean and prove their value to dieters. To do this, some manufacturers list the calories, proteins, carbohydrates, and fats in a single product serving. This is called a short nutrition list.

Others may use a longer nutrition list that gives the basic information in the short list, plus a chart on the U.S. Recommended Daily Allowances (RDAs). The U.S. RDAs show what percent of the daily recommended amounts of protein and certain vitamins and minerals you can get in a single serving.

HEALTH CLAIMS ON LABELS

In 1987, the FDA gave the green light to processors who wished to make health claims on their labels, provided that:

- The claim is truthful and not misleading.
- The claim is supported by valid, reliable, publicly available scientific evidence derived from well designed and conducted studies.
- The claim is consistent with generally recognized medical and nutritional principles for a sound total diet.
- The food is labeled in accordance with other relevant requirements.

The benefits of calcium, fiber, low fat, and so forth can now be used to sell products.

Some medical organizations, such as the American Heart Association, tried to establish a Consumer Health Information Program, in which three or four food categories would be designated and then marketers of food products in those categories would be asked to submit their products for healthfulness testing. Companies with products that won an American Heart Association seal of approval would then have been cleared to use that endorsement in advertising and labeling. The AHA would have used the money from fees paid by the food companies to finance educational advertising. The fees for each brand to participate in the Heart Guide would have ranged from ten thousand to forty thousand dollars to cover overhead and testing. The FDA, food processors, and some consumer groups objected to the program, and in 1990 the AHA was forced to drop its rating plans.[3]

The Procter and Gamble Company earlier received the seal of approval from the American Medical Women's Association (AMWA) for its calcium-fortified orange juice, Citrus Hill.® The AMWA charges companies twelve thousand dollars to apply for its endorsement. Procter and Gamble stopped advertising the endorsement of Citrus Hill but continues to use the seal. The endorsement didn't seem to convince anyone that its O.J. was better than others.[4]

In the meantime, the Mayo Clinic, which in the past has declined to use its name in any product endorsement, is getting prepared to do so. At this writing, the clinic is introducing a diet plan that recommends certain foods by brand name.[5]

Changes in regulations for food labeling are being crafted as this book is being written, and are expected to be in force in June 1991. These will be the first changes in the regulation of food labeling since the FDA spelled out what nutrition labels should state in 1973. Since then, reports from the Surgeon General of the Public Health Service, National Academy of Sciences, and others have stated that by changing diet, risks of certain diseases can be reduced.

The food industry has jumped on the bandwagon and many companies have issued a profusion of health claims on their products.

General Mills' Total Cereal, for example, has emblazoned across the front of the package "Meets all 7 food recommendations of the U.S. Surgeon General," is "calcium rich" and has "100 percent Daily Allowance of 12 Vitamins and Minerals."

The back of the package lists the Surgeon General's recommendations:

1. Reduce consumption of fat (especially saturated fat) and cholesterol.

2. Achieve and maintain a desirable body weight by choosing a dietary pattern in which energy (caloric) intake is consistent with energy expenditure.

3. Increase consumption of complex carbohydrates and fiber by choosing whole-grain foods and cereal products, vegetables, and fruits.

4. Reduce intake of sodium and limit the amount of salt added in food preparation at the table.

5. Those who are particularly vulnerable to dental cavities, especially children, should limit their consumption and frequency of use of foods high in sugars.

6. Adolescent girls and adult women should increase consumption of foods high in calcium, including low-fat dairy products.

7. Children, adolescents, and women of childbearing age should be sure to consume foods that are good sources of iron.

Next to the Surgeon General's recommendations, General Mills points out:

1. Total is a *no-cholesterol,* low-fat food.

2. Total has only 100 calories per ounce [does anyone eat one ounce of cereal?].

3. Total is made from whole-grain wheat and contains three grams of fiber per ounce.

4. Total, like many other breakfast cereals, is relatively low in sodium, having 200 mg per ounce.

5. Total is low in sugar, with 3 grams of sugar per ounce.

6. Total is the only "leading ready-to-eat" cereal that is a significant source of calcium.

7. Total is fortified with 100 percent of the U.S. RDA of iron.

General Mills offers to send a booklet based on the Surgeon General's Report. Such information could be beneficial to the consumer, but is General Mills stretching it with its claims for Total? One ounce of Nabisco's Cream of Wheat, for example, has no cholesterol or fat, no sugar, 80 mg of sodium, 100 calories, and no health claims, at least not at this writing. General Mills, on its Cheerios cereal box, claims "Lowest Sugar of the leading brands," one gram compared to Kellogg's Corn Flakes with two grams. Cheerios also touts its eight grams of oat bran and offers a book on the back of the box, "How to Lower Your Cholesterol and Beat the Odds of a Heart Attack."

While some senators and thirty-four state attorneys general are considering legislation to ban all health claims on food packages, the FDA is inclined to allow the following:

Fiber may reduce the risk of colon cancer and heart disease; low fat may reduce the risk of cancer and heart disease; low salt may reduce the risk of high blood pressure; and high calcium may help prevent the bone disease osteoporosis.[6]

What should you do? Educate yourself about the above recommendations by the FDA; recognize that food manufacturers want to sell you their products. You would have to eat a tremendous amount of bran cereal to lower your cholesterol. Cheerios, for example, has eight grams of oat bran, but to reduce your cholesterol 3 percent, you would need to eat thirty-five grams of oat bran.[7] If you ate enough cereal to lower your cholesterol 3 percent, not only would you be very full but you would have over 1,000 milligrams of sodium and 440 calories. Make a considered choice.

What about the traditional nutritional information on the food package?

CARBOHYDRATE INFORMATION

Many cereal manufacturers voluntarily supply this (per serving) information on a package's nutrition label panel. Information given includes:

Starch and Related Carbohydrates   00 grams
Sucrose and Other Sugars   00 grams
Total Carbohydrates   00 grams

To understand this, it pays to remember:

- 4 grams of sugar equal 1 teaspoon (12 grams = 1 tablespoon).
- 4 grams of carbohydrates are equal to 1 calorie.

This information makes it easy to figure out how much sugar is contained in each serving and the number of calories that are sugar-supplied.

BY ANY OTHER NAME

Certain product ingredients bear a variety of names that camou-
flage their identity and go undetected easily. Beware of the following ingredients if you are trying to cut down on them or cut them out
of your diet completely:

sodium	sweeteners	saturated fats
baking powder	dextrin	animal fat
baking soda	dextrose	butter
plain/flavored salt	fructose	coconut oil
self-rising flour	galactose	hydrogenated compounds with shortening
anything with sodium in the name	sucrose	palm oil
	glucose	palm-kernel oil
	lactose	
	maltose	

Also beware of these popular claims that may be seen on meat
and poultry products:

- "Natural" means that the meat or poultry product is minimally
  processed and that it contains no artificial flavors, preservatives, or colors.
- "Imitation" is used on products made to resemble, or substitute
  for, other products. "Imitation sausage," for instance, must
  appear on products that look like sausage but do not contain the
  specific ingredients required by USDA product standards.
- "Treated with Radiation." Some meats are treated with radiation to kill microorganisms. They must be labeled "treated with
  radiation" or "treated by irradiation," and the irradiation logo
  must be shown on the label.
- Salt claims. Various sodium claims appear on products with
  reduced sodium contents. These claims are based on the amount

of sodium in a serving size. The actual amount of sodium must be indicated on the label. Processors must use one of the following:

- "Sodium Free" or "Salt Free." Products must contain 5 milligrams (mg) or less of sodium per serving.
- "Very Low Sodium." Products must contain 35 mg or less of sodium per serving.
- "Low Sodium." Products must contain 140 mg or less of sodium per serving.
- "Unsalted" or "No Salt Added." Products were processed without salt. Caution: These products may contain other sources of sodium, such as monosodium glutamate.
- "Reduced Sodium." Product must contain at least 75 percent less sodium than does the traditional product.
- "Lower" or "Less Salt" or "Sodium." Product must contain at least 25 percent less sodium than does the traditional product.
- Fat claims that are used on products that are naturally low in fat or that have a reduced fat content. They are:
  - "Extra Lean." Products must contain 5 percent or less fat by weight. Actual amount of fat must be indicated on the label.
  - "Lean" and "Low Fat." Products must contain 10 percent or less fat. The amount of fat must be indicated on the label. Some products may be labeled "Lite."
  - "Lite," "Lighter," "Leaner," and "Lower Fat." Products must contain 25 percent less fat than do similar products on the market. "Lite" can have various meanings, including a reduction in the fat, calories, sodium, or breading of a product. Reading the label can help you choose the product you want.

STANDARDS OF COMPOSITION

Controlled by the USDA, these standards govern and define the amounts of cooked meat and poultry that processed products must contain. Simply put, these standards state how much chicken goes into the pot pie along with the peas and gravy. The manufacturers' compliance with these standards helps you when you shop for quality foods.

STANDARDS OF IDENTITY

Standard foods follow a defined recipe and need not list ingredients on the label. A standard of identity (recipe) describes the ingredients the food must contain if it is to be called by a particular name—for example, ketchup, mayonnaise, or ice cream. The FDA sets standards of identity, quality, and amount in containers to protect us from being defrauded by cheap substitutes or deceptive packaging. Some three hundred standards are in force, covering a wide array of foods. A standard of identity tells not only what ingredients *must* be in food, but also what other ingredients *may* be added.

FOOD GRADING

The USDA has established grades for more than three hundred different food products. *Grading is done voluntarily at the manufacturer's request (and expense) by a USDA inspector;* the product may then display the USDA grade symbol on the package. Lack of a symbol does not mean the product is substandard.

Unfortunately, these grades lack continuity among product categories (Grade AA is the highest grade for eggs; Grade A is the highest for milk), so the information they communicate is questionable. Plans have been proposed to update grading.

Meat and poultry must be inspected and must carry an inspection stamp whether they are fresh or processed and packaged.

If a food is to be combined with other ingredients (for instance, cereal with milk), nutrition information may also be given for the combination.

STATE-INSPECTED PRODUCTS

Some products are inspected by state-run inspection programs. State-inspected products must meet standards equal to those of the federal government. These products must show a state-inspection mark and can be sold only within that state.

UNITED STATES DEPARTMENT OF AGRICULTURE INSPECTION MARK

USDA inspectors check beef and poultry to ensure that safely prepared, properly labeled products reach consumers. The official USDA inspection mark or stamp means the product was inspected.

You can find the inspection stamp on processed meat, such as canned beef stew, and on processed poultry, such as chicken franks.

The stamped information includes the number of the plant in which the product was produced. The plant number is preceded by the letters "EST," for "establishment" on processed meats, and with the letter "P" on poultry. The plant number makes it easy for the USDA to refer to the plant that processed the product should a problem occur.

Although it is not part of the inspection information, the name and address of the producer is listed. This is the company you can contact if you have a problem with or question about the product. To help you, the company may ask specific information about the product, such as the lot or batch number, if it's included on the package, and the net weight.

The lot or batch number tells on what day and on what shift the products were produced. If the products are recalled from the market, the numbers identify the lots.

The net weight tells the weight of the contents inside the container. This figure must be on the label and can be shown in pounds or fluid ounces.

HANDLING INSTRUCTIONS

Following handling instructions is the best way to ensure that products remain safe to eat.

Today, the packaging of products that need refrigeration is similar to that of those products that can be stored on the shelf. Therefore, it is necessary to follow the directions on the label to make sure you handle the product properly.

All perishable products must give handling instructions, such as "Keep Frozen" or "Keep Refrigerated." Some meat and poultry products may be labeled "Ready-to-Eat" or "Fully Cooked," which means that no further cooking is necessary. Other product labels may have directions on how long and at what temperature to cook the product. These directions are not required, nor have they been verified by the USDA. When cooking instructions are not included on the label, your best bet is to closely follow a recipe and thoroughly cook the product.

WANT A DATE?

Do you ever look for a date on a package? Since more than half the food purchased today is processed, you should know if you are buying "freshness."

Since I first wrote *Poisons in Your Food,* more processors have moved toward open dating. You'll find on packages "Sell by May 29" or "Use by September 7" or "For Best Quality, Use by June 1992." Some two dozen states now require open dating, primarily on perishable foods such as milk and ice cream, packaged bread, frozen dough products, and processed meats such as cold cuts and sausages. Under federal law, infant formula must also carry an expiration date.

Many products have dates on them, even though dating is optional. The date stamped on product packages can indicate product freshness and can serve as a guide to safe storage time, provided you know how to use it.

What do these dates mean?

- The "sell by" date tells the last day the product should be sold. The "use by" date tells you how long the product will retain top eating quality after you buy it.
- Some products may have an "expiration date," which tells you the last day the food should be eaten or used.
- Canned and packaged foods have "pack" dates that tell you when the product was processed.
- For frozen-food producers, freshness dating is a guess because it is almost impossible to determine how carefully the product is

going to be handled after it leaves the plant. It might be defrosted and refrozen several times.

Food processors and retailers still have a variety of codes to inform retailers and distributors—but not customers—about the freshness of products in cans, jars, and packages. Usually, one of two possible coded dates is on the product—either the date on which the product was processed or the date on which it should be "pulled" from the shelf. Generally, highly perishable products are given pull dates. Some of the codes, however, require that you take along a pocket-size calendar and a pencil.

Food processors are often masters at making codes inconspicuous. On frozen-food packages, the dates are usually indented on the wrapper or the carton. These colorless indentations are most often found at one end of the package. Another method of dating frozen food involves putting a small letter or number on the food wrapper. It is not stamped, but is part of the printing on the wrapper. Cans have the code numbers embossed on one end of the can, usually the bottom. Boxes have either stamped or indented codes on one end of the package.

It would be impossible to give all the codes here, but most supermarkets keep a thick book of master codes in their offices. If you have no success in breaking the code of a particular product, and store personnel feign ignorance, ask to see the code book. If the store refuses, write to your congressman and send copies of your letter to your local newspaper, board of health, and to the manufacturer. Chances are, you will get quick action.

Notes

CHAPTER 1

1. R. E. Duggan and Keith Dawson, "Pesticides," a report on residues in food, U.S. Food and Drug Administration reports, *FDA Papers* 1, no. 5 (June 1967). Tom Bogaard, chemist and general manager, Kenya Pyrethrum Co., interview with author, January 1968. Dr. George Kupchik, director of environmental health, American Public Health Association, tape-recorded interview with author, February 26, 1968.

2. William E. Jennings, director of the Division of Meat Inspection of New York, *The National Provisioner*, April 20, 1963. Rodney E. Leonard, deputy assistant secretary, Consumer and Marketing Service, U.S. Department of Agriculture, November 9, 1967, Congressional Hearings on Meat Inspection, Washington, D.C.

3. Howard J. Sanders, "Food Additives," *Chemical and Engineering News,* October 17, 1966. *Changing Times,* May 1960.

4. W. C. Hueper, former chief of the Environmental Section, National Cancer Institute, and W. D. Conway, *Chemical Carinogenesis and Cancers* (Springfield, Ill.: C. C. Thomas, 1965), 645.

5. *Food Marketing Review,* 1987, U.S. Department of Agriculture, Economic Research Services, report no. 590, Washington, D.C., August 1988, 46.

6. *Regulating Pesticides in Food: The Delaney Paradox,* National Research Council Committee Report, National Academy of Sciences Press, Washington, D.C., May 20, 1988.

7. John W. Yunginger, M.D., et al., "Fatal Food-Induced Anaphylaxis," *Journal of the American Medical Association* 260, no. 10 (September 9, 1988): 1450–1452.

8. S. W. Lagakos, B. J. Wessen, and M. Zelen, "An Analysis of Contaminated Well Water and Health Effects in Woburn, Massachusetts," *Journal of the American Statistical Association* 81, no. 395 (September 1986): 583–596.

9. *Regulating Pesticides in Food.*

10. Frank E. Young, M.D., Ph.D., "FDA's Year of Foods," *An FDA Consumer Special Report, Safety First: Protecting America's Food Supply;* Young, personal communication with author and investigators at the Centers for Communicable Diseases, Atlanta, Ga., June 1989, 4–5

11. Young, ibid.

12. Dr. George Kupchick, taped interview with author, February 26, 1968; seven interviews with inspectors, caterers, and vending-machine operators in 1989, all of whom wish to remain anonymous.

13. "Food and Drug Administration: Laboratory Analysis of Product Samples Needs to Be More Timely," U.S. Congress GAO Report, September 1986; "Pesticides: Better Sampling and Enforcement Needed on Imported Foods," U.S. Congress GAO Report, April 1986.

14. James Brooker, director of the Division of Fisheries Inspection, personal communication with author, February 1971; H. R. Robinson, chairman, legislative committee, American Shrimp Association, New Orleans, U.S. Senate Hearings, Wholesale Fish and Fishery Products Act of 1969, July 1, 2, and 14, 1969.

15. *Fish & Seafood Facts and Figures,* National Fisheries Institute publication, Washington, D.C., 1988.

16. Testimony of the National Fisheries Institute, on H.R.3735, before the Subcommittee on Livestock, Dairy and Poultry of the Committee on Agriculture, March 24, 1988.

17. *Food Marketing Review,* 1987, p. 3; FDA, personal communication with author, Washington, D.C., 1988–1989; Food and Drug Administration Proposed Fiscal Year 1989 Budget, February 19, 1988; and Emil Corwin, press officer, Food and Drug Administration, personal communication with author, September 7, 1989.

18. "The Food and Drug Administration," *Journal of the American Medical Association* 262, no. 2 (July 14, 1989).

19. *Food Marketing Review,* 1987, 11.

20. Howard Bauman, Ph.D., vice president of Pillsbury Company, speech before National Conference on Food Protection, sponsored by the American Health Association, Denver, April 4–8, 1971.

21. Chris Lecos, "Of Microbes and Milk: Probing America's Worst *Salmonella* Outbreak," *FDA Consumer,* February 1986, 18–21.

22. Steven Ostrow, M.D., personal communication with author, June 1989.

23. Lynette D. Hazelton, "Fast Food and Mini-Marts Bite into Grocers," *New York Times,* June 18, 1989.

24. Robert Scheuplein, Ph.D., Office of Toxicological Sciences, Center for Food Safety, Food and Drug Administration, American Association for Advancement of Science, New Orleans, February 19, 1990; and personal communication with the author, April 16, 1990. (Extrapolated from both sources.)

25. Toxicity Testing Strategies to Determine Needs and Priorities, National Research Council (U.S.), National Academy of Sciences, Washington, D.C., 1987.

26. Linda Tollefson, "Monitoring Adverse Reactions to Food Additives in the U.S. Food and Drug Administration," *Regulatory Toxicology and Pharmacology* 8 (1988): 438–446.

27. Roger D. Middlekauf, partner in the law firm McKenna, Conner and

Cuneo, Washington, D.C., "Delaney Meets De Minimis," *Food Technology* 39, no. 11, November 1985, 62–69.

28. Sanford A. Miller, director, Center for Food Safety and Applied Nutrition, Food and Drug Administration, *Proceedings of the AILS International Symposium on Safety Assessment*, November 19–20, 1984, Tokyo, Japan, 60–68.

29. "Congress Eyes Major Rewrite of Nation's Food Safety Laws," *American Medical News*, June 24, 1983, 10.

30. U.S. Department of Agriculture, *The Yearbook of Agriculture*, 1966, Washington, D.C., 28.

31. Bernard Weiss, Ph.D., University of Rochester School of Medicine, *Nutrition Update* 1 (1983): 21–38; and Charles Vorhees and R. E. Butcher, *Developmental Toxicology*, ed. K. Snell (London: Croom Helm, 1982), 247–298.

32. M. R. Zavon, R. Tye, and L. Latoree, The Kettering Laboratory Department of Environmental Health, College of Medicine, University of Cincinnati, Cincinnati, Ohio, "Chlorinated Hydrocarbons Insecticide Content of the Neonate," *Annals of the New York Academy of Sciences* 160 (June 23, 1969): 196–200.

33. Rita Meyninger and Christopher Marlowe, "The Model Cleanup," *Civil Engineering*, May 1989.

34. *Essex County (N.J.) Medical Society Bulletin*, 1967.

35. Ibid.

CHAPTER 2

1. Karl H. Kolmeier and Edwin D. Bayrd, "Familial Leukemia: Report of an Instance and Review of the Literature," *Proceedings of the Staff Meetings of the Mayo Clinic* 38 (November 20, 1963).

2. *New York Times*, November 27, 1967.

3. American Academy of Pediatrics, "Environmental Hazards Center Attention on Children," Fact Sheet, 1989.

4. A. Blair and D. W. White, "Death Certificate Study of Leukemia Among Farmers from Wisconsin," *Journal of the National Cancer Institute* 66 (1981), 1027–1030.

5. K. Cantor, G. Everett, A. Blair, et al., "Farming and Non-Hodgkin's Lymphoma," *American Journal of Epidemiology* 122 (1985), 535.

6. W. A. Blattner, A. Blair, and T. J. Mason, "Multiple Myeloma in the United States, 1950–75." *Cancer* 48, 2547–2554.

7. "Farming and Cancer," Backgrounder from the National Cancer Institute, September 4, 1986, 1–10.

8. Philip Shabecoff, "EPA Proposing Quicker Action Against Suspect Farm Chemicals," *New York Times*, July 20, 1989, 1.

9. C. H. Hoffman and L. S. Henderson, "Protecting Our Food," *U.S. Yearbook of Agriculture*, 1966.

10. Michael Dover, *Technology Review*, November/December 1985, 53.

11. Keith Schneider, "Curbs on Deadly Insecticide Are Urged," *New York Times*, March 21, 1989, A16.

12. Ibid.

13. Irma West, M.D., "Pesticides as Contaminants," *Archives of Environmental Health* 9 (November 1964).

14. J. A. Venkat, et al., USDA, ARS, Beltsville Agricultural Research Center, Beltsville, Md., "Analysis of p-Nitrophenol in Fog," paper presented at the 198th American Chemical Society National Meeting, September 10–15, 1989, Miami, Fla.

15. Charlotte J. Schomburg, et al., USDA, ARS, Beltsville Agricultural Research Center, Beltsville, Md., and Department of Environmental Toxicology, University of California at Davis, paper presented at the 198th American Chemical Society National Meeting, September 10–15, 1989, Miami, Fla.

16. Lamont Cole, Ph.D., "Pesticides: A Hazard to Nature's Equilibrium," *American Journal of Public Health*, 54, no. 1 (January 1964): 30–31.

17. Keith Schneider, "Pesticide Barred in 70's Is Found to Taint Poultry," *New York Times*, March 16, 1989, A16.

18. Albert H. Meyerhoff, *New York Times*, May 26, 1987.

19. *Regulating Pesticides in Food: The Delaney Paradox*, National Research Council Committee Report, National Academy of Sciences Press, Washington, D.C., May 20, 1988.

20. West, "Pesticides As Contaminants."

21. *Medical World News*, June 1963.

22. *Poisoned Harvest: How to Protect Your Children Against Pesticides in Foods*, Natural Resources Defense Council, 1989, P.O. Box 96641, Washington, D.C., 20090.

23. Barry Meier, "Poison Produce: As Food Imports Rise, Consumers Face Peril from Use of Pesticides," *Wall Street Journal*, March 26, 1987, 1.

24. W. B. Deichmann, Ph.D., J. L. Radomski, Alberto Rey, department of pharmacology, University of Miami Medical School, "Retention of Pesticides in Human Adipose Tissue—Preliminary Report," *Industrial Medicine and Surgery* 37, no. 3 (March 1968): 218–219.

25. *Medical World News*, August 23, 1968; and S. Gerson, M. B. Shaw, and F. H. Shaw, Ph.D., University of Melbourne and Prince Henry Hospital, Melbourne, Australia, *Lancet* 1: 1,371–1,374.

26. Roger Lewin, *Science* 229 (4710) (July 19, 1985): 257–258.

27. "Residues in Foods—1987," Food and Drug Administration Pesticide Program, *Journal of the Association of Official Analytical Chemists*, November/December 1988, 8.

28. Cesar Chavez, "A Letter from Cesar Chavez," *Eating Clean*, Center for Study of Responsive Law (Washington, D.C., 1987), 143–145.

29. *Science News Letter* 91 (June 17, 1967).

30. "Residues in Foods—1987," 2.

31. Ibid.

32. "As Farm Workers Help Keep American Health, Illness May Be Their Harvest," Medical News & Perspectives, *Journal of the American Medical Association*, June 9, 1989, 3,207.

33. Marguerite L. Leng, North American Agricultural Products Department, The Dow Chemical Company, Midland, Mich., "Consequences of Reregistration on Existing Pesticides," paper presented at the 198th American Chemical Society National Meeting, September 10–15, 1989, Miami, Fla.

34. Philip Shabecoff, "E.P.A. Proposing Quicker Action Against Suspect Farm Chemicals," *New York Times,* July 20, 1989, 1.

35. "Food and Drug Administration: Laboratory Analysis of Product Samples Needs to Be More Timely," U.S. Congress GAO Report, September 1986; "Pesticides: Better Sampling and Enforcement Needed on Imported Foods," U.S. Congress GAO Report, April 1986.

36. "Residues in Food—1987," 9.

37. Ibid.

38. "EPA Urges Ban on Use of Cancer-linked Fungicide for 45 Crops in U.S.," Associated Press, December 5, 1989.

39. Shelley Hearne, Natural Resources Defense Council, 1984, "Harvest of Unknowns: Pesticide Contamination in Imported Foods," *Eating Clean,* Center for Study of Responsive Law, Washington, D.C.

40. Meier, "Poison Produce," 1.

41. Ibid.

42. Ibid.

43. Ibid.

44. "FSIS Monitoring and Controlling Pesticide Residues in Domestic Meat and Poultry," USDA Office of the Inspector General, 1988, Washington, D.C.

45. *Regulating Pesticides in Food.*

46. "EPA Clears New Pesticides Capable of Causing Cancer," *Wall Street Journal,* October 13, 1988, A12.

47. "The Pesticide Alarm," *Rutgers Magazine for Alumni and Friends,* April–June 1989, 8.

48. *Hawley's Condensed Chemical Dictionary,* 11th edition, edited by Richard Lewis Senior and N. Irving Sax (New York: Van Nostrand Reinhold, 1987), 127.

49. Bruce Ames and Lois Swirsky Gold, "Pesticides, Risk, and Applesauce," *Science,* May 10, 1989, 755–757.

50. H. Eric Semler, "Supermarkets Plan to Boycott Table Grapes," *New York Times,* June 29, 1989, B1.

51. Keith Schneider, "Food Industry Now Testing Crops for Pesticides to Calm Consumers," *New York Times,* March 17, 1989, B1.

52. Barry Thomas, Schering Agrochemicals Limited, United Kingdom, "Changes in European Regulations," paper presented at the 198th American Chemical Society National Meeting, September 10–15, 1989, Miami, Fla.

53. D. D. Kauffman, Soil-Microbial Systems Laboratory, USDA, ARS, Beltsville Agricultural Research Center, Beltsville, Md., "Enhanced Biodegradation of Pesticides in Soil: The Phenomenon and Its Possible Significance," paper presented at the 198th American Chemical Society National Meeting, September 10–15, 1989, Miami, Fla.; and Joel R. Coats and L. Somasundaram, department of entomology, Iowa State University, Ames, Iowa, "Influence of Pesticide Metabolites on the Development of Enhanced Microbial Degradation," paper presented at the 198th American Chemical Society National Meeting, September 10–15, 1989, Miami, Fla.

54. Philip Shavecoff, "100 Chemicals for Apples Add Up to Enigma on Safety," *New York Times,* February 5, 1989, 6.

55. Cathleen J. Somich, Mark Muldoon, and Philip C. Kearney, "Field Trials

Using Ozone and Biologically Active Soil As a Disposal Method for Pesticide Waste and Rinsate," paper presented at the 198th American Chemical Society National Meeting, September 10–15, 1989, Miami, Fla.

56. Richard Amerman, personal communication with author, September 6, 1989.

57. William Bowers, department of entomology, University of Arizona, Tucson, "Insecticidal Compounds from Plants," paper presented at the 198th American Chemical Society National Meeting, September 10–15, 1989, Miami, Fla.; and Horace Cutler, USDA, ARS, Athens, Ga., "Herbicidal Compounds in Plants," paper presented at the 198th American Chemical Society National Meeting, September 10–15, 1989, Miami, Fla.

58. R. C. Beier, U.S. Department of Agriculture, Veterinary Toxicology and Entomology Research Laboratory, College Station, Tex., paper presented at the 198th American Chemical Society National Meeting, September 10–15, 1989, Miami, Fla.

59. R. C. Beier, U.S. Dept. of Agriculture, ARS, Veterinary Toxicology and Entomology Research Laboratory, College Station, Tex., paper presented at the 198th American Chemical Society National Meeting, September 10–15, 1989, Miami, Fla.

60. Murray Blum et al., department of entomology, University of Georgia, Athens, and Laboratory of Chemistry, National Heart, Lung and Blood Institute, Bethesda, Md., "New Insect Repellents Derived from Insect Natural Products," paper presented at the 198th American Chemical Society National Meeting, September 10–15, 1989, Miami, Fla.

61. "Sex Attractants for Pest Control Need Faster Approval," *Science Feature Ideas from Cornell,* July 12, 1989.

62. Sue Shellenbarger, "Pest-fighting Wasps May Help U.S. Farmers," *Wall Street Journal,* July 6, 1989, B4.

63. R. C. Koestler, Pennwalt Corporation, Bryan, Tex., "Pesticide Microencapsulation—Past, Present and Future," paper presented at the 198th American Chemical Society National Meeting, September 10–15, 1989, Miami, Fla.

64. Kenneth A. Barton and Paul F. Umbeck, University Green, Middleton, Wisc., "Expression of Bacillus Thuringiensis Delta-Endotoxin in Commercial Crop Plants," paper presented at the 198th American Chemical Society National Meeting, September 10–15, 1989, Miami, Fla.

65. James McKinley, Jr., "Test of Genetically Altered Pesticide Allowed," *New York Times,* July 6, 1989, A13.

66. Keith Schneider, "Sheep Replacing Defoliants in Oregon," *New York Times,* July 2, 1989, 6.

67. Keith Schneider, "Big Farm Companies Try Hand at Organic Methods," *New York Times,* May 26, 1989, 1.

68. Owen Woodier, "Can't Keep 'Em Down in D.C. Once They've Seen This Farm," *New York Times,* July 19, 1989, C3.

69. Philip Gutis, "Judge Overturns Strict Rules on Telling Public of Pesticides," *New York Times,* May 12, 1989, B4.

70. Leslie Roberts, "A Corrosive Fight over California's Toxics Law," *Science,* January 20, 1989, 306–309.

71. Kings Supermarket, Short Hills, N.J., April 26, 1989.

CHAPTER 3

1. John W. Yunginger, M.D., et al., "Fatal Food-Induced Anaphylaxis," *Journal of the American Medical Association* 260, no. 10 (September 9, 1988): 1,450–1,452.

2. Ibid.

3. Case of Rita L. Don, M.D., 102 University Towers, 1900 N. Oregon St., El Paso, Tex. Given to author by Steven S. Lockey, M.D., 60 N. West End Ave., Lancaster, Pa., 1968.

4. *New York Times*, March 4, 1968.

5. A. M. Rulis and D. G. Hattan, "FDA's Priority-Based Assessment of Food Additives," *Regulatory Toxicology and Pharmacology* 5, 152–174 (1985) and personal communication with author, August 1988.

6. James L. Goddard, M.D., Food and Drug Administration commissioner, tape-recorded interview with author, May 1968.

7. Paul E. Johnson, "Health Aspects of Food Additives," *American Journal of Public Health* 56 (June 1966): 6.

8. Linda Grace, "There Are No Harmless Substances," *World Health*, April 1969, 20–22.

9. *Nutrition Action Health Letter*, May 1989, 13.

10. Deborah Mesce, "Cancer-Causing Dioxin Found in Paper Milk Cartons," Associated Press wire story, September 1, 1989.

11. *Adverse Reactions to Foods*, American Academy of Allergy and Immunology Committee on Adverse Reactions to Food and National Institute of Allergy and Infectious Diseases, NIH Publication no. 84-2442, July 1984, p. 79.

12. Ibid.

13. Howard G. Rapport, M.D., *Journal of Asthma Research* 5 (September 1967).

14. Department of Health and Human Services, Food and Drug Administration, Quarterly Report on Adverse Reactions Associated with Sulfiting Agents, April 3, 1989, Washington, D.C.

15. Ibid.

16. "FDA Chief Reportedly Opposes Wider Sulfite Curbs," Associated Press wire story, June 21, 1989.

17. *Code of Federal Regulations: Food and Drug Administration Food and Drugs Parts 100–169, Revised*, April 1, 1988, Washington, D.C.

18. Joseph B. Miller, M.D., "Hidden Food Ingredients, Chemical Food Additives and Incomplete Food Labels," *Annals of Allergy* 41 (August 1978): 93–97.

19. Peter Greenwald, M.D., director, Division of Cancer Prevention Control, National Cancer Institute, "Nutrition and Cancer," statement, National Cancer Institute, May 1986, based on testimony given November 13, 1985, before the U.S. Senate Committee on Labor and Human Resources.

20. *Inspection Operations Manual*, FDA, April 6, 1987.

21. Ruth Winter, *Cancer-Causing Agents* (New York: Crown, 1979), 147.

22. *Federal Register*, June 16, 1986.

23. Richard Oberfield, M.D., "Liver Cancer," *CA—A Cancer Journal for Clinicians*, July/August 1989, 16.

24. Dr. William Wardell, director of the Center for the Study of Drug Development, University of Rochester, speaking at a symposium, Public Issues and Private Medicine, December 6, 1978, in Philadelphia.

25. Ibid.

26. "Aflatoxin in Corn," *FDA Consumer,* May 1989, 2.

27. Ibid.

28. Ibid.

29. Hearings before a Subcommittee of the Committee on Government Operations, House of Representatives, June 10, 1970, Washington, D.C.

30. Ibid.

31. Ibid.

32. Ibid.

33. Ibid.

34. Ibid.

35. Senator Warren Magnuson to Secretary of Health, Education, and Welfare Elliot L. Richardson, December 22, 1970.

36. Personal communication with Dr. Paul LaChance, professor of Food Science, Rutgers University, New Brunswick, New Jersey.

37. *Medical Tribune,* July 6, 1970, 11.

38. G. A. Bray in "Obesity in America" from *Obesity in America,* G. A. Bray, Editor, NIH Publication no. 79-359, 1–19, National Institutes of Health, 1979.

39. "Aspartame: Review of Safety Issues," American Council on Scientific Affairs, *Journal of the American Medical Association* 254 (1985): 400–402.

40. Department of Health and Human Services, Food and Drug Administration, Quarterly Report on Adverse Reactions Associated with Aspartame Ingestion," April 3, 1989, Washington, D.C.

41. Linda Tollefson, "Monitoring Adverse Reactions to Food Additives in the U.S. Food and Drug Administration," *Regulatory Toxicology and Pharmacology* 8 (1988): 438–446.

42. "Aspartame Critics Persist: Recommended Avoidance During Pregnancy," *Medical World News,* December 12, 1986, 21.

43. Department of Health and Human Services Quarterly Report on Aspartame.

44. P. S. Spencer, D. N. Roy, A. Ludoph, J. Hugon, et al., "Lathyrism: Evidence for a Role of the Neuroexcitatory Amino Acid BOAA," *Lancet,* November 8, 1986, 10,066–10,067.

45. Erik Eckolm, "Monosodium Glutamate Still a Mystery," *New York Times,* April 23, 1986, C1.

46. Ruth Winter, *A Consumer's Dictionary of Food Additives,* 3d ed., rev. (New York: Crown, 1989), 162.

47. "Neurotoxins As Food Ingredients," John Olney, Dennis Choi, Claude de Montigny, Social Issues Roundtable: Neurotoxins in Our Daily Diet, presented at Society for Neuroscience 19th Annual Meeting, Phoenix, Arizona, October 31, 1989.

48. Ibid.

49. Marilyn Smith Claggett, M.S., R.D., "Nutritional Factors Relevant to Alzheimer's Disease," *Journal of the American Dietetic Association* 89 (March 1989): 392–396.

50. Tollefson, "Monitoring Adverse Reactions to Food Additives."

51. "FDA Clamps Down on Red Dye Additive," Associated Press, Washington, D.C., January 30, 1990.

52. Arthur Winter, M.D., and Ruth Winter, *Eat Right Be Bright* (New York: St. Martin's, 1988), 82.

53. W. C. Hueper, former chief of the Environmental Section, National Cancer Institute, and W. D. Conway, *Chemical Carcinogenesis and Cancers* (Springfield, Ill.: C. C. Thomas, 1965), 654.

54. Winter, *A Consumer's Dictionary*, 219.

55. "Juiceless Apple Juice Convictions Overturned," *FDA Consumer*, June 1989, 3.

56. *Modern Medicine*, January 1, 1968.

CHAPTER 4

1. *The Effects on Human Health of Subtherapeutic Use of Antimicrobials in Animal Feeds* (Washington, D.C.: National Academy Press, 1980).

2. Dr. Gerald Guest, director of the FDA's Center for Veterinary Medicine, *FDA Consumer*, November, 1988, 28.

3. "Food Additives Status List Updated to January 1, 1988," Inspection Operations manual transmittal notice, FDA.

4. Ibid.

5. T. C. Byerly, "Use of Human Subjects in Safety Evaluation of Food Chemicals," National Academy of Sciences, 1967.

6. Murray C. Zimmerman, *Archives of Dermatology* 79 (January 1959).

7. Konard Wicker, Ph.D., Robert E. Reisman, M.D., and Carl E. Arbesman, M.D., "Allergic Reactions to Penicillin Present in Milk," *Journal of the American Medical Association* 208, no. 1 (April 7, 1969): 143.

8. Alexander Fisher, *Contact Dermatitis*, 3d ed. (Philadelphia: Lea & Febiger, 1986), 200–201.

9. *Physicians Desk Reference*, 43rd ed. (Oradell, New Jersey: Medical Economics Press, 1989), 2,100.

10. *Drugs in Livestock Feed*, vol. 1, Technical Reports, Office of Technical Assessment, July 12, 1979.

11. *Physicians Desk Reference*, 1,485.

12. "Human Health Risks with the Subtherapeutic Use of Penicillin or Tetracyclines in Animal Feed," Washington, D.C., April 1989.

13. Abe Brown, "What You Need to Know About Salmonella," *Current Health*, September 1986, 10.

14. Larry Thompson, "Tracking Bacteria Back to the Farm," *Washington Post Health* March 10, 1987, 18.

15. "Serving up Salmonella for Dinner," *U.S. News & World Report*, March 9, 1987, 60–61.

16. *FDA Consumer*, June 1988, 2.

17. Frank E. Young, M.D., Ph.D., "A Lesson in Industry Education: Keeping Drug Residues Out of Milk," *FDA Consumer*, March 1989, 7.

18. Keith Schneider, "FDA Plans Action on an Animal Drug: Sulfamethazine Contaminates Milk and Pork Supplies," *New York Times*, November 5, 1989, 1.

19. Bruce Ingersoll, "Milk Is Found Tainted With a Range of Drugs Farmers Give Cattle," *Wall Street Journal,* December 29, 1989, 1.

20. WCBS-TV News Department, broadcasts on February 5 and 6, 1990.

21. "FDA Survey Gives Milk Supply a Clean Bill of Health in 13 Major U.S. Cities," *Star-Ledger,* February 6, 1990, 3.

22. "Science Doesn't Support European Beef Ban," *FDA Consumer,* April 1989, 2.

23. Bruce Ingersoll, "Supermarket Chains Spurn Milk Products from Growth Hormone Treated Cows," *Wall Street Journal,* August 24, 1989, B2.

24. "Labor Saving Slow Release Bovine Somatotropin Tested Successfully at Cornell," Cornell University press release, Ithaca, N.Y., June 14, 1989.

25. Ingersoll, "Supermarket Chains," p. B2.

26. Keith Schneider, "FDA Accused of Improper Ties in Review of Drug for Milk Cows," *New York Times,* January 12, 1990, A2.

27. Hormone to boost milk production seen meeting public resistance," *American Medical News,* October 20, 1989, 39.

28. Ingersoll, "Supermarket Chains," p. B2.

29. Bill Rados, "Keeping Our Food Safe from Animal Drugs," *FDA Consumer Special Report,* November 1988, 28.

30. Ibid.

31. Ibid.

32. Ibid.

33. Keith Schneider, "Tainted Milk and Meat Raise Vigilance," *New York Times,* May 11, 1989, A18.

34. Ibid.

35. Senator Walter F. Mondale to author, February 14, 1968.

36. Ibid.

37. Bruce Ingersoll, "Inspection Cuts at Meat Plants Placed on Hold," *Wall Street Journal,* April 5, 1989, A4.

38. USDA press release, February 2, 1988.

39. "Chicken Industry Called Unsafe and Uncontrolled," *New York Times,* July 30, 1989, 24.

40. Ibid.

41. *Poultry Inspection: The Basis for a Risk-Assessment Approach,* National Research Council Committee report (Washington, D.C.: National Academy Press, 1987).

42. Ibid.

43. Richard Whiting, USDA Microbiological Food Safety Laboratory, Philadelphia, personal communication with author, September 5, 1989.

44. Report of the National Research Council of the National Academy of Sciences, *Designing Foods: Animal Product Options in the Marketplace,* April 5, 1988, Washington, D.C.

CHAPTER 5

1. Murray Wittner, M.D., Ph.D., et al., "Eustrongylidiasis—A Parasitic Infection Acquired by Eating Sushi," *New England Journal of Medicine* (April 27, 1989): 1,124–1,129.

2. Steven Ostroff, M.D., epidemiologist, Communicable Disease Center, Atlanta, Ga., personal communication with author, July 1989.

3. Vern Modeland, "Fishing for Facts on Fish Safety," *FDA Consumer*, February 1989, 16.

4. Michele Manges, "Trying to Lure Back Seafood Consumers," *Wall Street Journal*, June 27, 1989, B1.

5. Werner A. Janssen and Caldwell D. Meyers, *Science* 159 (February 2, 1968).

6. Editorial, *Archives of Environmental Health* 2 (May 1966).

7. Herbert L. DuPont, M.D., "Consumption of Raw Shellfish: Is the Risk Now Unacceptable?," *New England Journal of Medicine* 314, no. 11 (March 13, 1986): 707–708.

8. Guy Sterling, "Four Charged in Illegal Clam Dealing," Newark *Star-Ledger*, July 23, 1989, 44.

9. DuPont, "Consumption of Raw Shellfish," 707–708.

10. Morbidity and Mortality Weekly Report, Centers for Disease Control, March 10, 1989, vol. 38, no. 9, 140–142.

11. *Merck Manual*, 15th ed., Robert Berkow, M.D., ed. (Rahway, New Jersey: Merck & Company, 1987), 787.

12. "The Raw Truth About Fish," *Emergency Medicine*, July 15, 1986, 42.

13. Gordon Bishop, "Scientist Urges Mid-Atlantic States to Unite on Preserving Coastal Waters," *Newark Star-Ledger*. June 16, 1989, 35.

14. "Highly Invasive New Bacterium Isolated from U.S. East Coast Waters," *Journal of the American Medical Association* 251, no 3 (January 20, 1984): 323.

15. Carol Ballentine, "Weighing the Risks of the Raw Bar," *FDA Consumer*, September 1986, 23.

16. "Infectious and Parasitic Diseases," *Merck Manual*, 15th ed., Robert Berkow, M.D., ed. (Rahway, N.J.: Merck & Company, 1987), 197–234.

17. Dale Blumenthal, "Minute Shrimp," *FDA Consumer*, May 1989, 29.

18. "Gastroenteritis: Infective and Toxic," *Merck Manual*, 15th ed., Robert Berkow, M.D., ed. (Rahway, N.J., Merck & Company, 1987), 780.

19. "The Raw Truth About Fish," 30–50.

20. Philip Shabecoff, "U.S. Toxic Chemicals Are Imperiling Aquatic Life," *New York Times*, June 14, 1989, A24.

21. William Schmidt, "Toxic Risk of Fish in Lake Michigan Is Assessed," *New York Times*, June 29, 1989, A20.

22. Nancy Hicks, "Mercury Detective," *New York Times*, May 21, 1971, 31.

23. Dixie Farley, "Chemicals We'd Rather Dine Without," *FDA Consumer 2*, November 1988, 23.

24. *New York Times*, March 14, 1989, 2.

25. Farley, "Chemicals We'd Rather Dine Without," *FDA Consumer 1*, September 1988, 15.

26. Ibid.

27. Thomas Morgan, "Court Allows Fishermen's Suit on PCBs in Hudson," *New York Times*, March 20, 1989, A4.

28. Keith Schneider, "Puget Sound Fish Farms Challenged," *New York Times*, July 8, 1989, 6.

29. Vern Modeland, "FDA Nets Makers of Unapproved Fish Drugs," *FDA Consumer*, September 1988, 38–39.

30. *NFI Position on Seafood Inspection,* statement, June 1, 1989, Washington, D.C.

31. "Hazardous Fish: The Raw Facts," Public Voice for Food, *Eating Clean,* 1988, 59.

32. *Nation's Restaurant News* 23, no. 15 (April 10, 1989): 2.

33. Lee J. Weddig, National Fisheries Institute, speech before National Academy of Sciences, January 31, 1989.

34. "Visual Inspection of Seafood Ineffective, Cornell Expert Tells U.S. Subcommittee," Cornell University News Release, February 7, 1990, Washington, D.C.

35. Weddig, ibid.

CHAPTER 6

1. Chris Lecos, "The Public Health Threat of Food-Borne Diarrheal Disease," *FDA Consumer,* November 1985, 19–22.

2. "Salmonella Types, Hazards on Rise," *American Medical News,* May 12, 1989, 18.

3. Ibid.

4. Ibid.

5. Lecos, "Public Health Threat."

6. H. P. R. Seeliger, "Listeriosis—History and Actual Developments," *Infection* 16 (1988), supplement 2.

7. Ibid., p. S.80–S.83.

8. Chris Lecos, "Of Microbes and Milk: Probing America's Worst *Salmonella* Outbreak," *FDA Consumer,* February 1986, 18–20.

9. Lawrence Altman, "Questions Raised on Role of Cheese in Salmonella," *New York Times,* January 24, 1990, A10.

10. Lecos, "Of Microbes and Milk."

11. *FDA Drug Bulletin,* February 1989, 6.

12. "Update: *Salmonella enteritidis* infections and Grade A Shell Eggs—United States, 1989," Centers for Disease Control Morbidity and Mortality Weekly Report, January 5, 1990, 38, nos. 51 & 52.

13. James Goddard, M.D., Commissioner of U.S. Food and Drug Administration, "Incident at Selby Junior High," *Nutrition Today,* September 1967.

14. Congressional Hearing on Food Irradiation, 1987.

15. University of Michigan News Service, October 9, 1968.

16. Dennis Blakeslee, feature story, University of Wisconsin News Service, December 10, 1963.

17. Ralph W. Johnson, M.S., John Feldman, A.B., and Rosemary Sullivan, B.S., *Public Health Reports,* July 1963. The names of the victims are fictitious.

18. Ibid.

19. Miscellaneous press reports July 3–6, 1971.

20. *FDA Bulletin,* April 1989.

21. Editorial, *Journal of the American Medical Association* 194, no. 5 (November 1, 1965).

22. "Foul Flying Subs," *FDA Consumer,* July–August 1989, 34–35.

23. Miscellaneous news coverage; "PHS Traces Epidemic of Fatal Diarrhea," *Medical World News,* June 4, 1965.

24. Steve Ostroff, M.D., medical epidemiologist, Centers for Disease Control, Enteric Division, Atlanta, Ga., personal communication with author, June 29, 1989.

25. Timothy Cover, M.D., and Robert C. Aber, M.D., "Yersinia Enterocolitica," *New England Jounal of Medicine,* July 6, 1989, 16–21.

26. Ibid.

27. *Merck Manual,* 15th ed., Robert Berkow, M.D., ed. (Rahway, N.J.: Merck & Company, 1987), 204–205.

28. Dean O. Cliver, Ph.D., "Food-associated Viruses," *Health Laboratory Science* 4, no. 4 (October 1967).

29. Edward Richardson, Jr., M.D., "Toxoplasmosis: The Time Has Come," *New England Journal of Medicine,* February 4, 1988, 313–316.

30. *Merck Manual,* 109.

CHAPTER 7

1. Mike Kelly, "As the Worm Turns," *Bergen (N.J.) Record,* November 17, 1988.

2. S. W. Lagakos, B. J. Wessen, and M. Zelen, "An Analysis of Contaminated Well Water and Health Effects in Woburn, Massachusetts," *Journal of the American Statistical Association* 81, no. 395 (September 1986): 583–596.

3. Ibid.

4. Robert Hanley, "Women's Leukemia Rate Higher in 4 New Jersey Towns," *New York Times,* December 13, 1987, 64.

5. Interim Report on Ground Water Contamination, House Committee on Government Operations, September 30, 1980.

6. J. Scott Orr, "Jersey Ranks No. 20 on Toxic Pollutants List," *Newark Star-Ledger,* June 20, 1989, 6.

7. Marvin Zeldin, "Our Drinking Water: A Threatened Resource," Public Affairs Pamphlet no. 613, Public Affairs Committee, New York, 1983.

8. Rita Meyninger and Christopher Marlowe, "The Model Cleanup," *Civil Engineering,* May 1989.

9. Luther Terry, M.D., surgeon general, U.S. Public Health Service, *The Week,* December 3, 1961.

10. J. Raloff, "No Threshold to Lead's Learning Effect," *Science News* 131 (June 13, 1987): 374.

11. "Fetal Lead Exposure Said to Retard Learning," *New York Times,* April 23, 1987, A22.

12. "Schools Warned of Lead in Water Fountains," Associated Press, Washington, D.C., April 11, 1989.

13. Jack Winter, Jayson Water Systems, Union, N.J., personal communication with author, August 15, 1989.

14. "Aluminum in Water Tied to Alzheimer's," *American Medical News,* March 3, 1989, 2.

15. "New Study Suggests Water Chlorination Linked to Bladder Cancer Risk," statement, National Cancer Institute, Office of Cancer Communications, December 1987.
16. The National Toxicology Program Study of Chronic Toxicity and Carcinogenicity of Sodium Fluoride Report, January 24, 1990, Washington, D.C.
17. Tom Johnson, "State Test Reveals Traces of Toxic Chemicals in 89 Drinking Water Systems," *Newark Star-Ledger,* March 22, 1985, 10.
18. Howard Earl, "Water Pollution: That Dirty Mess," *Today's Health,* March 1966.
19. Hunter Comly, M.D., *Journal of the American Medical Association,* January 29, 1945, 112–116.
20. John Lukens, M.D., "The Legacy of Well-Water Methemoglobinemia," *Journal of the American Medical Association* 257, no. 20 (May 22/29, 1987): 2,793–2,797.
21. *The Merck Manual,* 15th ed. Robert Berkow, M.D., ed. (Rahway, N.J.: Merck & Company, 1987), 213.
22. Edward Hayes, M.D., et al., "Large Community Outbreak of Cryptosporidiosis Due to Contamination of a Filtered Public Water Supply," *New England Journal of Medicine* 320 (May 25, 1989): 1,372–1,376.
23. Jane Brody, "The Appearance of Clean Water May Be Deceiving; An Elusive Parasite Can Cause Severe Diarrhea," *New York Times,* October 27, 1988, C12.
24. *Merck Manual.*
25. Luther Terry, M.D., *This Week.*
26. Tom Johnson, "Clean Water Won't Be Cheap as State Aims to Keep It Safe," *Newark Star-Ledger,* May 16, 1989, 1.
27. Betty H. Olson, Ph.D., University of California, "The Safety of Our Drinking Water," *New England Journal of Medicine* 320, no. 21 (May 25, 1989): 1,413–1,414.
28. Philip Shabecoff, "E.P.A. Adopts Stiffer Regulations to Protect Drinking Water Supply," *New York Times,* June 23, 1989, All.
29. Ibid., C1.
30. Tom Johnson, "Pollution Settlement Provides Water Study Aid," the Sunday (Newark) *Star-Ledger,* March 6, 1988, 50.

CHAPTER 8

1. *Food Service Industry, 1987 in Review,* National Restaurant Association. *Food Marketing Review,* USDA Research Service and Agricultural Economic Report, no. 590, August 1988.
2. Charles W. Felix, NPH, material for information kit on Food Handler Testing, Educational Testing Services, Princeton, N.J., 1985.
3. Center for Disease Control, Atlanta, Ga.
4. Aaron Haskins, M.D., Health Officer, Newark, N.J., "Physical Examination of Food Handlers Is Not a Useful Requirement," *Public Health News,* New Jersey State Department of Health, June 1967, and personal communication with author, July 1968.

5. *Make a S.A.F.E. Choice: A Sanitary Assessment of Food Environment: A New Approach to Restaurant Self-Inspection,* National Restaurant Association, Washington, D.C., 1987, 7.

6. Ibid.

7. Ibid., 16–17.

8. Pat Silvers, Educational Testing Service, Princeton, N.J., personal communication with author, August 30, 1989.

9. "From Hand to Mouth," U.S. Department of Health, Education, and Welfare, Public Health Service Publication no. 281.

10. Ibid.

11. S. R. Anderson, "Assessment of the Health Risks and Handling of Products Used in Food Service Establishments," *Journal of Environmental Health,* April 1985, 200–201.

12. *Make a S.A.F.E. Choice,* 1.

13. USDA Agricultural Research Service, "New & Improved Products," July 12, 1988: Statistical Government Publication.

14. William Clinge, tape-recorded interview with author, July 1968.

15. Dr. George Kupchik, director of environmetal health, American Public Health Association, tape-recorded interview with author, February 26, 1968.

16. Kathleen, Irwin, M.D., Jane Ballard, M.D., John Grendon, D.V.M., M.P.H., and John Kobayashi, M.D., M.P.H., "Results of Routine Restaurant Inspections Can Predict Outbreaks of Foodborne Illness: The Seattle–King County Experience," *American Journal of Public Health* 79, May 1989, no. 5, 586–590.

17. Samuel Leff, "Corruption in the Kitchen: A Health Inspector's Inside Story," *New York Magazine,* Oct. 17, 1988, 39–45.

18. Bea Hayton, "Salad Bars: As Good As They Look?," *Current Health* 2, September 1987, 14–16.

19. Jay McDaniel, "Two More Hospitalized from Tainted Church Dinner," *Newark Star-Ledger,* January 17, 1989, 2.

20. *Food Service Sanitation Manual, 1962,* Public Health Service publication no. 934.

21. David E. Hartley, "Vending Self-Regulation Protects Foods, Public Health," *Journal of Environmental Health* 45, no. 6 (May/June 1983): 292–294.

22. Michael Jacobson, "Let People Know What They Are Eating," *New York Times,* January 12, 1986, B1.

23. Ruth Winter, "Taking the Weight Off Business Dining," *Success,* February 1984, 52.

24. "On Dealing with Diarrhea Abroad," *Emergency Medicine,* November 30, 1985, 91–107.

CHAPTER 9

1. *Food Marketing Review,* United States Department of Agriculture, Economic Research Service, Agriculture and Economic Report, no. 590, August 1988.

2. Ibid.

3. Mark Clements, "Who Shops and Who Cooks," *Parade,* October 25, 1987, 12–13.

4. Sue Sellenbarger, "A Peeling Project Bears Fruit," *Wall Street Journal,* July 6, 1989, B1.

5. *Food Marketing Review,* 1988, 11.

6. Abraham Wolman, "Man and His Changing Environment," *Journal of Public Health,* November 1961.

7. Judann Dagnoil and Julie Erickson, "Grocery Retailers Get Tougher," *Advertising Age,* May 15, 1989, 4.

8. Ibid.

9. Laynette D. Hazelton, "Fast Food and Mini-Marts Bite into Grocers," *New York Times,* June 18, 1989, C2

10. Pat Terry, "Retailers Delight in Their Delis," *Advertising Age,* May 9, 1989, S6.

11. March 1968.

12. Lisa H. Towle, "What's New in Snack Food," *New York Times,* December 6, 1987, C2.

13. Alix M. Freedman, "As 'Fresh Refrigerated' Foods Gain Favor, Concerns About Safety Rise," *Wall Street Journal,* section 2, March 11, 1988, 1.

14. Ibid.

15. Ibid.

16. Ibid.

17. Barbara Toman, "Will U.S. Warm to Refrigerated Dishes?," *Wall Street Journal,* August 18, 1989, B12.

18. "Frozen Fruits, Vegetables and Precooked Frozen Foods," *Recommended Methods for the Microbiological Examination of Foods,* J. M. Sharf, ed. (American Public Health Association, 1967), March/October 1987.

19. George P. Larrick, former commissioner, U.S. Food and Drug Administration, speech delivered before National Association of Frozen Food Packers, Chicago, Ill., March 20, 1964.

20. Grace M. Urrows, "Food Preservation by Irradiation," U.S. Atomic Energy Commission, Division of Technology Information, April 1968.

21. "Frozen Fruits, Vegetables," 65.

22. *Food Facts from Rutgers University,* press release, New Brunswick, N.J., January/February 1968.

23. Ed Fitch, "Scouts Agree: It's Hot If It's Microwaveable," *Advertising Age,* May 9, 1988, S16.

24. Summary of paper by Barbara Miller, Dwight Miller, and Stanley Billedeau of the National Center for Toxicological Research in Jefferson, Ark., presented at the 194th national meeting of the American Chemical Society before the Division of Agricultural and Food Chemistry in the New Orleans Hilton, August 31, 1989.

25. "Food Preservation by Irradiation."

26. In May 1986, the Health and Energy Institute and the Environmental Policy Institute—two public interest groups concerned about the health effects of radiation—petitioned the FDA to revoke its food irradiation regulation and hold a public hearing. Bills have also been introduced in the Senate and House of Representatives calling for more research on irradiated foods before radiation regulations go

into effect. The Senate Bill, introduced by Senator George Mitchell (D, Maine), is S. 461. The House Bill, introduced by Representative Douglas Bosco (D, California), is H.R. 956.

27. Dr. Richard D. Holsten, Cornell University doctoral thesis, 1965.

28. Dennis Burkitt and H. C. Trowell, "Refined Carbohydrate Foods and Disease," Academic Press, London and New York, 1975.

29. *Consumer Reports,* February 1967, 64.

CHAPTER 10

1. *Journal of the American Medical Association,* November 18, 1961.

2. Color Additives Amendment, 17.

3. "Problems in the Evaluation of Carcinogenic Hazards from the Use of Food Additives," Food Protection Committee, Food and Nutrition Board, National Academy of Sciences, December 1959.

4. Sandford A. Miller, "The United States of America—Risk Assessment and U.S. Food Safety Policy," *Safety Assessment,* November 19–20, 1984, 60–68.

5. Linda Tollefson, D.V.M., M.P.H., chief, Clinical Nutrition Assessment Section, Center for Food Safety and Applied Nutrition, personal communication with author, June 2, 1989.

6. Linda Tollefson, "Monitoring Adverse Reactions to Food Additives in the U.S. Food and Drug Administration," *Regulatory Toxicology and Pharmacology* 8, 1988, 438–446.

7. Milton Z. Nichaman, M.D., D.S., and R. Sue McPherson, M.S., "Estimating Prevalence of Adverse Reactions to Foods: Principles and Constraints," *Journal of Allergy Clinical Immunology,* July 1986, 148–154.

8. Peter Greenwald, M.D., Dr. PH (Doctor of Public Health), director, Division of Cancer Prevention and Control, statement released by the National Cancer Institute, May 1986.

9. Pennington Associates, "CIIT, Founded by Chemical Industry, Is a Unique Toxicology Research Facility" (Pennington Associates, Raleigh, N.C.), April 29, 1987, 1–14.

10. Ibid.

11. Arthur Winter, M.D., and Ruth Winter, M.S., *Eat Right Be Bright* (New York: St. Martin's Press, 1988), 173–74.

12. "FDA Clamps Down on Red Dye Additive," Associated Press, Washington, D.C., January 30, 1990.

13. Thomas H. Maugh II, "How Many Chemicals Are There?," *Science,* April 15, 1983, 293.

14. A Strategy for a Livable Environment, report to the Secretary of Health, Education, and Welfare by the Task Force on Environmental Health and Related Problems, June 1967.

15. Adverse Reactions to Food, American Academy of Allergy and Immunology Committee on Adverse Reactions to Foods, National Institute of Allergy and Infectious Diseases, NIH Publication no. 84–2442, July 1984, 105.

16. Sushma Palmer, Sc.D., and Susan Berkow, Ph.D., "Nutrition Education in American Medical Schools," *Nutrition Today,* January/February 1986, 5–7.

CHAPTER 12

1. Denise Cabrera, "Law Makers Want to Shed Light on Food Labels," Associated Press, Washington, D.C., July 28, 1989.

2. How Nutritious Is It?," United States Department of Agriculture press release, May 29, 1987, Washington, D.C.

3. " 'Heart Guide' Food-Rating Program Attracts 114 Applications as Controversy Continues," *Journal of the American Medical Association* 262, no. 24, December 22/29, 1989, 3388.

4. Janet Meyers, "Dairy Industry Aims to Beat FDA on Labels," *Advertising Age,* 2–3.

5. Richard Gibson, "Mayo Clinic Diet Lists Food Brands," *Wall Street Journal,* February 2, 1990.

6. Philip J. Hilts, "FDA Acts to Limit Food Health Claims," *New York Times,* December 15, 1989, D17.

7. *Nutrition Action Healthletter,* Center for Science in the Public Interest, Washington, D.C., 1990.

Index

A

Ostroff, Steven, (Centers for Disease Control), 121, 171
Oxytetracycline, in animal feed, 93, 95
Oysters, 122–124

P

Packaging, migration of chemicals from, 60
PAFA. *See* Priority Based Assessment of Food Additives.
Palm oil, 282
Palm-kernel oil, 282
Paralytic shellfish poisoning (PSP), 128–129
Parkinsonism, and paraquat, 24
Parsley, 32, 35
PBBs (polybrominated biphenyls), in animal feed, 105–108
PCBs (polychlorinated biphenyls), 139
Peanuts/peanut oil, as hidden additive, 63
Penicillin, 9, 93–94
Pesticides, 45
  and cancer, 1
  natural, 44
  substitutes for, 42–43

Pharmacologic food reactions, 61
Phenoxy herbicides, 14
Potassium bromate, 73
Potassium nitrite. *See* Nitrates and nitrites.
Poultry:
  disease contracted from, 115, 160
  handling of, 160
  inspection of, 111–113
Precooked frozen foods, 244
Priority Based Assessment of Food Additives (PAFA), 254
Processing aids, in foods, 57, 59
Promoters, of cancer, 256
Ptomaine poisoning, 165–166
Public Citizen Health Research, 275
Public Voice for Food, 275, 277
Public Health Service. *See* United States Public Health Service.

R

Rapport, Howard G., 65
Raw fish, 120
Rector, Denise, 223
Red No. 2, 73